IMMEDIATE IMPLANT PLACEMENT

AF595410

Dr. Aadarsh Dhan

Dr. Hiroj Bagde

Dr. Aniket Sharan

Dr. Bhawna Shyamsukha

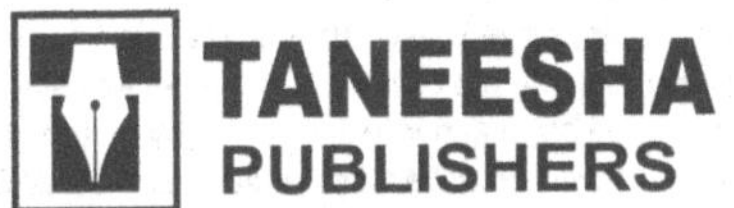

Title : Immediate Implant Placement

Author : Dr. Aadarsh Dhan, Dr. Hiroj Bagde,
Dr. Aniket Sharan, Dr. Bhawna Shyamsukha

Edition : First (August, 2024)

ISBN : 9788197792724

Copyright © 2024, All Rights Reserved by Author

Published by

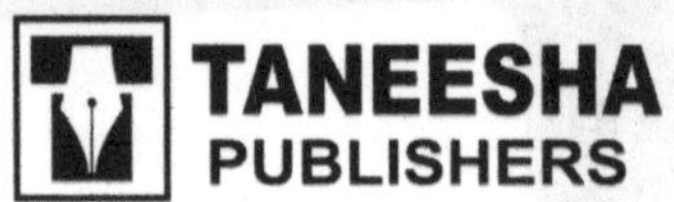

A Venture by -
PRACHI DIGITAL PUBLICATION

Regd. Add.: 254, Khuriyakhatta No. 10, Bindukhatta,
Lalkuan, Nainital - 262402, Uttarakhand, India
Website : www.taneeshapublishers.in
E-mail : taneeshapublishers@gmail.com
Phone : +91 845481 2712, +91 976041 7980

Printed by :
Manipal Technologies Limited, Bengaluru - 560001, Karnataka

COPYRIGHT NOTICE & PUBLISHER DISCLAIMER

Copyright rights of this book including compositions, descriptions, statements, opinions included in this book are reserved by the author, so no any part of this book shall be reproduced partially electronic or mechanical (including film, serial, photographic, without the written permission of the author Recording, any newspaper, magazine, literary portal news portal, blog or translation into another language) in any manner whatsoever without written permission from the author, except in the case of brief quotations embodied in critical articles and reviews. If a person or institution attempts to do so, they will be responsible for the legal action.

Disclaimer : This book has been published with all efforts taken to make the material error-free after the consent of the author. However, the author and the publisher do not assume and hereby disclaim any liability to any party for any loss, damage, or disruption caused by errors or omissions, whether such errors or omissions result from negligence, or any other cause. While every effort has been made to avoid any mistake or omission, this publication is being sold on the condition and understanding that neither the author nor the publishers or printers would be liable in any manner to any person by reason of any mistake or omission in this publication or for any action taken or omitted to be taken or advice rendered or accepted on the basis of this work. For any defect in printing or binding, the publisher will be liable only to replace the defective copy by another copy of this book then available through the same seller or distributor where purchased it.

CONTENTS

INTRODUCTION

Restoring teeth to their ideal state regarding form, comfort, appearance, function, speech & general health is goal of modern dentistry. This can be accomplished by treating dental caries or by replacing several missing teeth, fixed, removable, or implant-supported prostheses being most common options.[1] Patients who are completely or partially edentulous can now have restorations done on them thanks to placement of endosseous implants.[2] Word "immediate" appears in the implant literature almost every day, albeit it's frequently used ambiguously. When the phrase was first used, it referred to the procedure of placing implant during extracting tooth. It is currently used for refering to the immediate insertion of a provisional restoration into a socket or onto a healed bone complex on an implant that has just been positioned. The phrase is also used when a provisional restoration is positioned on an implant that is placed right away and the restoration needs to accept functional occlusal loads right away.[3]

In 1952, Per-Ingvar Brånemark observed that titanium implants and bone can osseointegrate.[4] When placing dental implants, his original protocol called for six to eight months of recovery after extraction, sterile conditions utilizing a mucobuccal flap, and a 2-stage process of placing machined titanium implants followed by three to six months of stress-free healing for osseointegration to occur. A course of therapy will last for a whole year or more. Employing a two-phase method, such as Brånemark's protocol, gives rise to further worries regarding alveolar bone volume loss, extended treatment durations, prolonged edentulism, further surgical procedures, and psychological impacts on patient. The alveolar ridge experiences bone remodelling after tooth extraction, especially during first year.[4]

Advancements in technology and surgical techniques have led to significant alterations to original implant protocol, resulting in predictable and promising outcomes.[1] One of these protocols is placing an immediate implant, which involves placing it into recent extraction sockets right after tooth removal.[1] Immediate implant placement can described by placing an implant immediately following extraction during & after ,which often needs a bone grafting technique for addressing any defects around the implant.[5] Concept of IIP first described by Schulte & Heimke in 1976, later reintroduced by Lazzara in 1989 through case reports.[1]

The morphology of extraction socket influences clinician's choice of flap design, need for bone grafting, implant size selection & whether to non-submerge/submerge implant while healing.[1] In 1993, D.A. Gelb reported a collection of 50 persistent cases with 98% survival rate, which validated the immediate placement protocol.[6] In general dentistry practices today, immediate implant placements are more common, particularly for single missing teeth, as patients find the conventional six-month healing period following extraction to be less convenient. As a result, in implant dentistry, timing of placement has become very essential.[1]

HISTORY

There is an informative and remarkable history behind the invention of dental implants. Since the beginning of time, individuals have replaced missing teeth in one way or another using dental implants. Egyptians tried using gold ligature wire for supporting teeth which were affected by periodontal process around 2500 BC. Their manuscript contains many intriguing variables to toothaches. To restore human oral function, Etruscans created personalized soldered gold bands from animals and replaced human teeth with oxen bones around 500 BC. These creative people created a fixed bridge around 300 AD using cleverly carved ivory teeth held together by gold wire. The gold wire was utilized by the Phoenicians to stabilize teeth which were impacted by periodontal disease. The first dental implants were said to have been made by Mayan people, which adept at replacing mandibular teeth with pieces of shell around 600 AD.[7] In an experiment, a rooster's comb was used to receive an immature tooth, as Dr. Hunter proposed transplanting human teeth into another person. He saw an amazing thing happen: tooth firmly attached itself to rooster's comb, & blood vessels developed directly in tooth pulp.[8]

An Iridio-platinum cylinder with a 24-gauge hollow lattice that was soldered with 24-karat gold implanted by **Dr. EJ Greenfield** in 1913 as prosthetic root, and it was designed for "fit exactly circular incision made in patient's jaw." [9] It was also believed that the Strock brothers were the ones who successfully inserted first endosteal (in bone) implant. **Dr. P.B. Adams** received a patent of 1938 for cylindrical endosseous implant including healing cap and smooth gingival collar.

Both inside and outside implant were threaded.[10] Owing to the efforts of **Dr. Leonard Linkow**, the idea of immediate implantation got started years ago. He created vent implant, first self-tapping endosseous root-form implant, in 1963. In the end, technique that was chosen called for loading these implants right away with temporary acrylic bridges or overdentures.[11]

To enable implant insertion and achieving optimal fit, French physician **Dr. Raphaël Cherchève** magnify spiral design through incorporating burs. The subperiosteal implant created by Dahl in Sweden 1940s as implant study progressed. In 1960s, designs became more diverse. Double-helical spiral implant made of cobalt & chromium created by Dr. Cherchève. It is now accepted that blade implant is an endosseous implant. Later, in the middle of the 1960s, **Dr. Sandhaus** created a soldered bone screw that was primarily composed of aluminium.[12] **Dr. P. Brånemark** debuted 2-stage threaded titanium root-form implant in 1978, also evaluated & created approach called fixtures that used just titanium screws.[13]

Two other pioneers in field of contemporary implantology were Swiss Physicians **Dr. Straumann & Dr. Schroder**. They conducted experiments on metals used in orthopaedic surgery which aid with creation of dental implants.[14] The prosthetic consideration, surface roughness, design, ease of insertion in cost,bone & long-term success of an endosseous implant system were main determinants in which system was selected over another.

Early in the 1980s, **Dr. Tatum** unveiled Omni R implant, which featured titanium alloy horizontal fins. Shortly after, in the 1980s, **Dr. Driskell** unveiled Stryker "root-form" endosseous implant. This device comes in two varieties: a titanium alloy version and a hydroxyapatite-coated version.[12]

RECOGNITION OF IMPLANT DENTISTRY

There was virtually little research on dental implants in 1972. With regard to dental implants, the American Dental Association (ADA) adopted a cautious stance and assigned Natellia et al. to investigate viability of dental implants for clinical usage. According to survey, "there is limited approval for implants by profession, which was matter of international concern." "Endosseous implants should not be recommended during routine clinical use," American Dental Association stated in 1974, adding that they "should be considered as novel procedure phase or need of continuing scientific inquiry." Based on a few specific requirements and warnings, the ADA's Council on Dental Materials and Devices provisionally approved endosseous dental implants in the early 1980s. The Biotes (Nobelpharama, Gothenburg, Sweden) was the only endosseous implant approved by the ADA in 1986.[15]

Use of dental implants has expanded significantly in current year to raise standard in living for people. About 5.5 million dental implants were cultivated in the US alone in 2006; by 2018, total value of US dental implants was estimated to be around $5 trillion (Alani et al., 2014).[16] Development in different biocompatible materials, technical frameworks and components may expand the range of bio-based applications for dental implants; however, certain problems still exist (Bhat and Kumar, 2013).[17]The overall amount of time from extraction to final restoration was shortened by improvements in implant surface technology and higher patient expectations. The concept of instantaneous implant insertion (IIP) at shorter intervals originated from this tendency. Socket anatomy can impede the ideal three-dimensional positioning of IIP, leading to a less acceptable result. While main implant stability is critical success factor for implantation placement procedures (IIPs), crestal bone level (CBL) variations around IIP are influenced by a number of other parameters as well.[18]

History of implantology at the time of Mayan civilization[15]

Investigators	Place	Period	Implant like substances
Popenoe, an archaeologist (1931)	Playa-de-los Muertos in the Ulna River valley of Honduras in middle America	600 A.D.	Artificial tooth carved from a dark stone—mandibular left lateral incisors
		800 A.D.	Three tooth-shaped pieces of shell—missing lower incisors—alloplastic biomaterials

History of Implantology - depend on eras[15]

Periods	Time
A.D 1000	Ancient year
1000-1800	Medieval period
1801-1910	Foundational period
1911-1935	Premodern era
1936-1978	Dawn of the modern era (pre-Brånemark era)
1978-1998	Scientific basis of implantology (Brånemark era)
1998-present era	Post-Brånemark era — immediate loading

CLASSIFICATION OF IMPLANTS

Depending on penetration into tissues:[19]

a. Mucosal implants-Palatal inserts:

b. Subperiosteal implants:

c. Trans-osteal implants:

d. Endosteal implants:

e. Blade implants:

f. Pins:

g. Disk implants:

h. Root form:

i. Endodontic implant/endodontic stabilizers:

Depending on Macroscopic Body Design of Implant:[19]

a. Cylindrical. (Hollow; Straumann –ITI, full; Kirsch- IMZ): They are either gently and pushed knocked into place.

b. Screw-shaped (tapered) implants: They are either self-tapped into prepared dental implant site or inserted following tapping of bone with a screw tap.

c. Blade form (Linkow)

d. Pins.

e. Endodontic stabilizers.

Depending on implant design or number of surgeries required:[19]

a. Submerged / Two-stage implant

b. Non-submerged / one stage

Depending on surface of implant:[19]

a. Smooth surface

b. Machined surface

c. Textured surface

d. Coated surface

Depending on implant-abutment interface of implant:[19]

a. External hex

b. Internal hex

Depending on implant materials used:[19]

Materials used for fabrication of dental implants can be divided in 2 ways:

Depending upon a chemical point of view; they are of 3 main groups

a. Metallic implants: Titanium, stainless steel, chromium cobalt.

b. Ceramics.

c. Polymers.

d. Miscellaneous: Carbon compound

Depending on type of biological response:[19]

It is based on response created after implantation & host tissue reaction in long term to implant.

3 major types of biodynamic activity are,

a. Bio-tolerant

b. Bioinert

c. Bioactive

Biodynamic activity	***Chemical composition***		
	Metals	**Ceramics**	**Polymers**
Biotolerant	Gold Cobalt-chromium alloys Stainless steel		Polyethylene Polyamide Polymethylmetha crylate Polytetrafluroeth

	Zirconium Niobium Tantalum		ylene Polyurethane
Bio-inert	Commercially pure titanium Titanium alloy (Ti-6Al-4V)	Aluminium oxide Zirconium oxide Poly-ether-ether-ketone	
Bioactive		Hydroxyapatite Tricalcium phosphate Tetracalcium phosphate Calcium pyrophosphate Fluorapatite Brushite Carbon-silicon Bioglass	

Based on the material used for implant production:[19]

1. Titanium and its alloys
2. Tantalum
3. Ceramics
4. Zirconia
5. Polymer
6. Poly-ether-ether-ketone (PEEK)

7. Newer biomaterials:
8. Ni-free Ti-based BMG alloys

Based on width of implant:[19]

- Narrow diameter Implant: ≤3.75 mm
- Conventional diameter : >3.75 mm but less than 4.5 mm
- Wide diameter: >5 mm.
- In a systematic review, **Javed** & **Romanos** resulted that long-term survival of implants in posterior maxilla was secondarily impacted by diameter.

Implant timing classification table. (Chen and Buser)[20]

Class	Definition	Advantages	Disadvantages
Type I	Implant placement as a part of same surgical procedure and *immediately* following extraction.	• Reduced number of surgical procedures and overall treatment time • Optimal availability of existing bone	• Site morphology may complicate optimal placement and anchorage • Thin tissue phenotype can compromise optimal outcome • Potential lack of keratinized mucosa for flap adaptation • Adjunctive surgical procedures can be needed • *Technique-sensitive*
Type II	*Complete soft tissue coverage* of socket (4–8 weeks)	• Increased soft tissue area & volume facilitate soft tissue flap management	• Site morphology may complicate optimal placement or anchorage • Increased treatment time • Varying amounts of

		• Allows assessment in resolution of local pathology	resorption in socket walls • Adjunctive surgical procedures may be required • Technique-sensitive
Type III	*Substantial bone fill* of socket (12–16 weeks)	• Substantial bone fill of socket facilitates implant placement • Mature soft tissues facilitate flap management	• Increased treatment time • Adjunctive surgical procedures may be needed • Varying amounts of resorption in socket walls
Type IV	*Healed site* (>6months)	• Clinically healed ridge • Mature soft tissues facilitate flap management	• Increased treatment time • Adjunctive surgical procedures may be required • Large variation in available bone volume

CLASSIFICATION OF IMPLANT PLACEMENT

1. Wilson & Weber (1998) – Implant Placement[21]

1	Immediate	Same day of extraction
2	Recent	30-60 days after extraction (Soft tissue healing)
3	Delayed	Following hard tissue maturation
4	Mature	6 months to years after extraction

2. **Mayfield et al. (1999)** [21]

Immediate	Same day of extraction
Delayed	42 – 70 days after extraction
Late	6 months after extraction

Esposito et al. Classified implants according to the Osseointegration Concept:[22]

a. Biological
b. Mechanical
c. Iatrogenic
d. Inadequate patient education

CLASSIFICATION OF IMMEDIATE IMPLANT PLACEMENT SITES[23]

Class I	- Buccal bone Intact - Thick gingival biotype - **Flapless Implant placement**
Class II	- Buccal bone Intact - Thin, scalloped gingival biotype - **Immediate implant placement and connective tissue graft or staged CTG.**
Class III	- Buccal bone is Lost **IIP+ GBR+ bone grafts + CTG.** - Based on degree of compromises of buccal plate, Case is alternatively handled with **staged approach.** - Indication for IIP is **limited**
Class IV	- Buccal bone is Severely compromised - **IIP in remaining palatal bone.** - Results in **significantly off Axial Implant placement.** - So, implant should be **delayed (Type IV)** If implant is placed Immediately Implant inclines towards buccal & will result in **Significant esthetic compromise**.

Bone Classification Schemes Related to Implant Dentistry

Linkow & **Chercheve,**[24] 1970, classified bone density in 3 categories:

- **Class I bone structure**: This ideal bone type consists of evenly spaced trabeculae with small cancellated spaces.
- **Class II bone structure**: Bone has slightly larger cancellated spaces with less uniformity of osseous pattern.
- **Class III bone structure**: Large, marrow-filled spaces exist in between one trabeculae.

Lekholm and Zarb[25] 1985 classified bone density using radiographs in 4 bone types depending on trabecular versus cortical bone amount.

- **Type 1** - composed of homogenous compact bone.
- **Type 2** - thick layer with compact bone surrounding a core of dense trabecular bone.
- **Type 3** - thin layer with cortical bone surrounding dense trabecular of favourable strength.
- **Type 4** - thin layer with cortical surrounding a core of low-density trabecular bone.

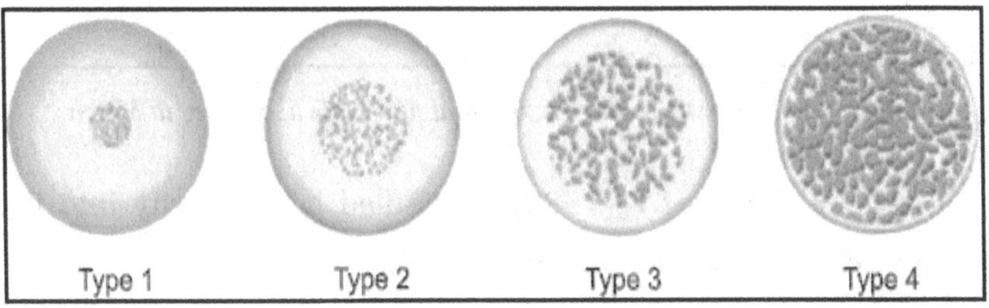

Fig.1 - Bone types classified according to Lekholm and Zarb based on the amount of cortical versus trabecular bone.

Misch Bone Density Classification Scheme (1988,1993) [26,27]

Bone	Density Description	Tactile Analog	Typical Anatomic Location
D1	Dense cortical	Oak or maple	Anterior mandible

		wood	
D2	Porous cortical and coarse trabecular	White pine or spruce wood	Anterior mandible Posterior mandible Anterior maxilla
D3	Porous cortical and fine trabecular	Balsa wood	Anterior maxilla Posterior maxilla Posterior mandible
D4	Fine trabecular	Styrofoam	Posterior maxilla Anterior maxilla
D5	Osteoid	Soft Styrofoam	Poorly mineralized bone graft

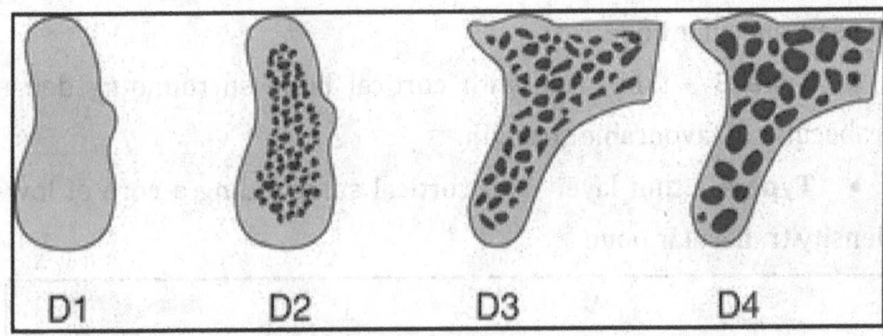

Fig.2 - Bone density in the maxilla and mandible according to Misch

Misch CE, Kircos LT (1999)[28] classified bone density into five groups depending on number of Hounsfield units (HU).

Type	**Hounsfield units (HU) [Density]**	**Region**
D1	greater than 1250 HU	anterior mandible, buccal shelf, and mid-palatal region
D2	850–1250 HU	anterior maxilla, mid-palatal

		region and posterior mandible
D3	350–850 HU	posterior maxilla & mandible
D4	150–350 HU	tuberosity region
D5	less than 150 HU	

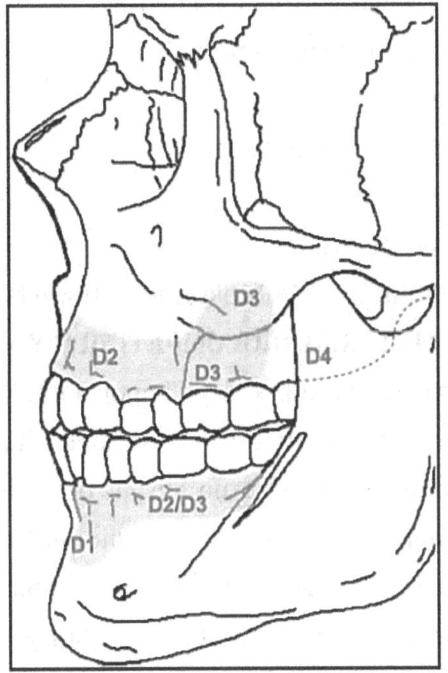

Fig.3 - Bone density in the maxilla and mandible according to Misch and Kircos

FACTORS ACCOUNTING FOR SUCCESSFUL OSSEOINTEGRATION

Primary and secondary elements that lead to effective osseointegration have several causes. For an implanted device to establish a dependable, long-term osseous anchoring, six distinct ones are known to be crucial. Factors included are:

Implant Material Biocompatibility.

1) Implant Design.
2) Implant Surface modification.
3) State Of Host Bed.
4) Surgical Considerations.
5) Loading Conditions.[29] (Albrektsson T, Albrektsson B)

1. IMPLANT MATERIAL BIOCOMPATIBILITY

Material's biocompatibility is important & predictor of osseointegration, which was important for establishing Stable fixation to direct bone-implant contact & no fibrous tissue at interface. Pure Titanium (Ti) widely used orthopedic metallic implant material which are highly biocompatible, good corrosion resistance, no toxicity on fibroblast and macrophages, lack of inflammatory response in peri-implant tissues, & its surface is composed of an oxide layer which can recover itself by reoxidation when damaged.[30] (Dimitriou R)

2. IMPLANT DESIGN

Earlier implant body design was decided based on ease of surgical placing implant. Various implant body designs can be used.

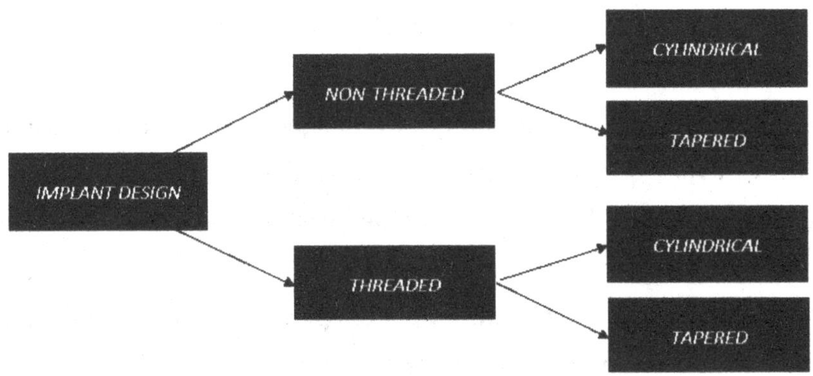

Cylindrical non-threaded implant design has convenience in surgical implantations, nevertheless. Contact between implant and bone exposed with much greater shear forces. It has low risk of pressure necrosis, no need for bone tap, also 1st stage cover screw is placed as no rotational force requiring for inserting implant.

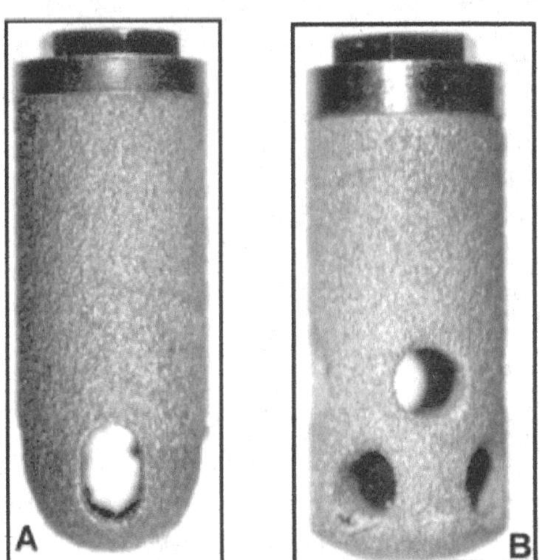

Fig.4 - Non – Threaded Implants

I. **Tapered non-threaded implant design** provides ease of implant placement. Though non-threaded provides component of compressive load delivered to bone-implant interface, based taper degree. They are easiest to place and have a high initial success rate.[31] (Yadav P)

II. **Cylindrical threaded implant design** requires a bone tap and care to avoid pressure necrosis. However, there was less implant failure and crestal bone due to fatigue overload as compared to that of non-threaded implants.

III. **Tapered threaded implant design** also requires a bone tap and care to avoid pressure necrosis. Placement of the implant is easier than with the cylindrical threaded design. The crestal bone loss and implant failure because of fatigue overload is least as forces are here more compressive than shear. A threaded implant has better primary stability than a press-fit implant.[32] (McGlumphy).

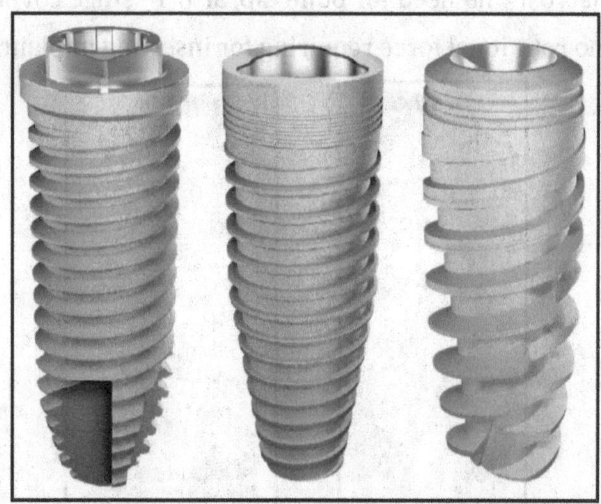

Fig.5 - Threaded Implants

THREAD GEOMETRY AND FUNCTIONAL SURFACE AREA

Threads on an implant body are designed to:

- Maximize initial fixation and bone contact

- Enhance surface area, &
- Facilitate the dissipation of loads at bone-implant interface.[32]

Functional surface area per unit length of implant can modified with three thread geometry parameters:

- Thread pitch
- Thread shape
- Thread depth

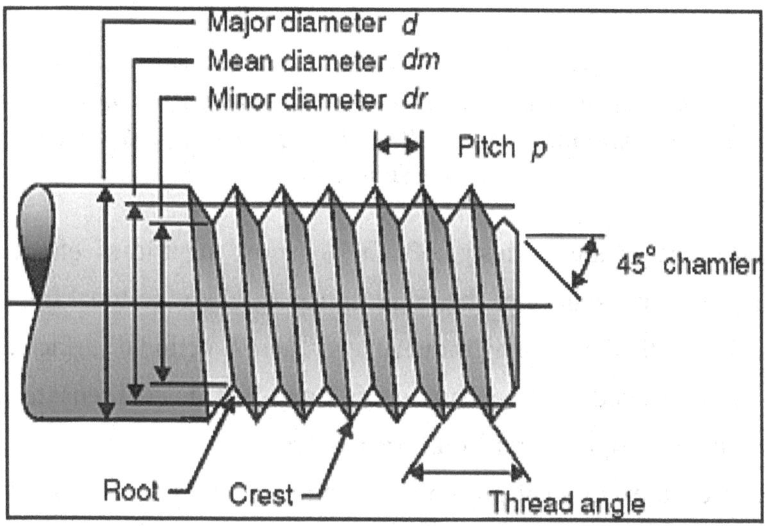

Fig. 6 - Parameters of an implant that may alter the functional surface area. Three of these include thread pitch, thread shape, and thread depth.

THREAD PITCH

Thread pitch defined as distance measured parallel between adjacent form features of an implant. Threads per unit length is length for threaded portion in implant body divided by pitch. Smaller or finer pitch, greater number of threads on body. This leads to increased surface area per unit length.[31]

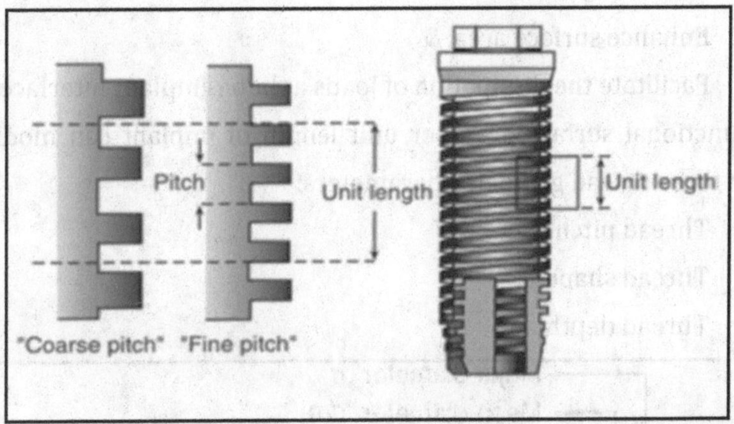

Fig. 7 - The implant on the right has a smaller thread pitch and greater surface area, whereas the implant on the left has the largest thread pitch and the least overall surface area.

Amongst variables design, Pitch has most significant effect for changing surface area of threaded. In cases where an ideal implant length is difficult to plan without surgery, here functional surface area can be improved by increasing no. of threads. This compensates for the reduced height dimension.[33] **(Rasmusson L)**

The ease of surgical placement of an implant is also affected by thread number. Fewer the threads easier it is for inserting implant. As dense bone difficult to bone tap the fewer number of threads Improves the ease of implant placement.[34] **(Misch CE)**

➢ **THREAD SHAPE**

Thread shapes in dental implant designs include:

- o V-shaped
- o Square
- o Buttress
- o Reverse buttress

V-shaped thread has a face angle of 30 degrees off long axis. This leads to an increased amount of tensile and shear loads. This is the most common thread design used for implants.

The **square thread** is perpendicular to the long axis. It provides optimized surface area for intrusive & compressive load transmission. It refers as power thread in engineering. The occlusal loads which are directed in axial direction along implant body may be compressive at bone interface.[31] **(Yadav P)**

Buttress thread shape optimized for pullout loads. The force transfer mechanism of buttress thread shape design to bone is similar to that of V-thread design.

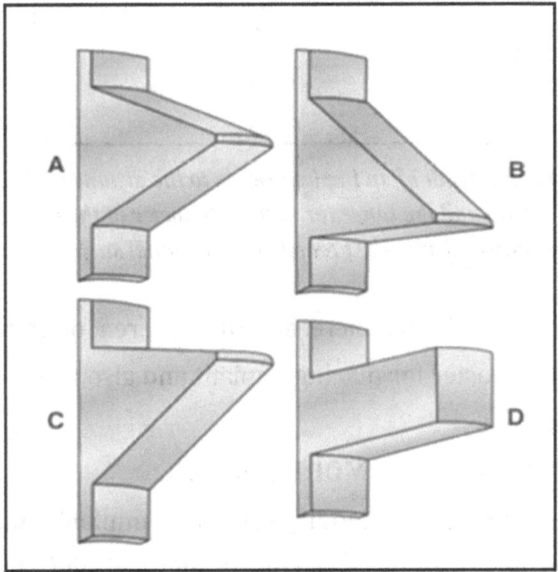

Fig.8 - The four basic thread shapes for implant design include:(A) V-thread, (B) buttress thread, (C) reverse buttress thread, and (D) square thread.

➢ THREAD DEPTH

Thread depth is distance between major & minor diameter of thread.

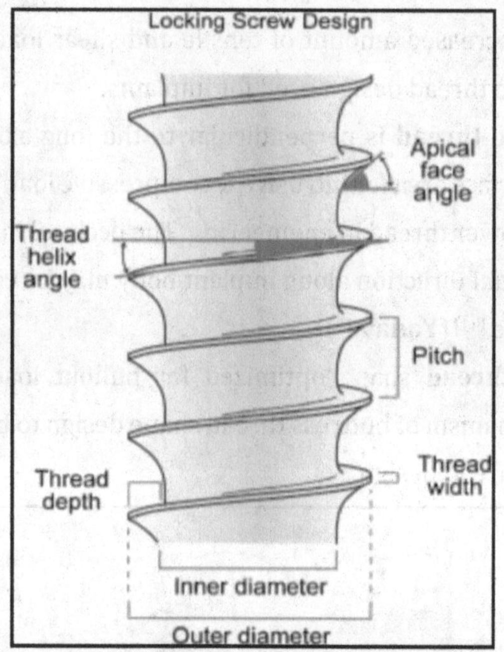

Fig. 9 - The thread depth of an implant refers to the distance between the outer (or major) diameter and the inner (or minor) diameter of the thread. The deeper the thread depth, the greater the functional surface area.

Greater thread depth, increase surface area of implant. When shallow will be easier for placing implant and also less likely tapping of bone is needed.

3. IMPLANT SURFACE MODIFICATION

The techniques used to modify surface of implants may generally divided into 3 categories: mechanical, physical and chemical. It is possible for modifying morphology, structure, and surface chemistry of implants using these various techniques. The primary goal of procedures is improving bio-mechanical characteristics of implant, involving improving wear and corrosion resistance, enhancing osseointegration by stimulating bone growth, and removing surface impurities.

1. **Mechanical methods:** It includes blasting, grinding, machining, & polishing. This technique involving physical treatment generally leads to smooth and rough surface that modify proliferation, differentiation and adhesion of cells.
2. **Chemical methods:** surface modification of titanium & its alloys by chemical treatment depends on reactions occurring at interface between titanium or solution. Its modifications comprise treatment with hydrogen peroxide, acids or base, sol-gel, and anodization and chemical vapour deposition. It has been widely applied to alter surface composition, roughness & increasing wettability/surface energy.
3. **Physical methods**: These include sputtering, plasma spraying involves atmospheric plasma spraying , vacuum plasma spraying & ion deposition which are used for creating titanium & CaP coatings on surfaces of titanium implants.

The method can also be classified as Additive and Subtractive.[35] Additive methods employed treatment in which other materials are added to surface, either superficial or integrated. Whereas, removal of surface material by mechanical methods involving grinding, shaping/removing, machining, & blasting to create roughness is included in subtractive methods.[36]

Machined

It is milled, turned,or polished, minimally rough, with surface area roughness (Sa) value 0.3—1.0 lm which was designed by manufacturing tools used, lubricant,implant material, & speed at which it is machined.[37]

Sandblasting

Bombardment with titanium surfaces of granules in variable diameter oxides like zirconium, titanium, aluminum oxide, & silicon carbide.[38] Resorbable blast media (RBM): bone-compatible material is used as blasting media for etching implant like Hydroxyapatite (HA) and tricalcium phosphate.[39]

Acid Etched

In order to enhance the characteristics of titanium & its alloys, demonstrated by Wen et al., this procedure is typically used in conjunction with other treatment techniques to remove oxide and contaminants for providing clean, consistent surface finishes. It was observed that using an alkaline solution and (HCl+H2 SO4) increases the bioactivity of Ti alloy.[40]

Alkaline Etched

The production of titanium nanostructures that extend from its surface is catalyzed by a sodium hydroxide (NaOH) treatment. Handling Heat treatment at 600°C transforms sodium titanate hydrogel layer into amorphous layer using a NaOH solution. A layer permits deposition of HA. Similar characteristics have also been seen with other metals, like aluminum and zirconium.[41]

Dual acid Etching

Double acid etching treats surface with chemicals and acid in sequence or a combination comprising both. It aims to produce cavities at submicron and nanometer scales as well as increase overlapping nano roughness. Second-acid etching aimed for improving specific surface area & nano roughness in comparison for single-acid etching.[42]

Laser Etching

It is a noncontact therapy for which implant surface not

contaminated with blasting media. Substrate material vaporizes and forms a crater. Furthermore, laser etching is more convenient method in controlling micro-topography of implant surface and enhances biocompatibility of implant surface.[43]

Grit Blasting

Abrasive blasting, often known as grit blasting, is another technique used to produce surface topographies on implant surfaces. In this, it is either rapidly suspended in a liquid or pelted with hard, dry particles. For grit blasting titanium, a variety of ceramic particle types, such as silica, alumina, etc., in various sizes can be utilized.[44]

Anodization

It goes through an electrochemical process called anodic oxidation in an electrolyte, which produces a microstructure surface with open holes size of micrometers. Phosphoric acid is used as the electrolyte and an implant passed current through to create surface oxide. For a better biological impact, anodized implant surfaces combine regulated oxide texture and porosity.[45]

Plasma Coating

Particles, titanium, and hydroxyapatite are projected onto surface using a plasma torch heated to extremely high temperatures in process known as plasma spraying. On the surface, particles condense and combine to form a coat. Smoother implants have not shown as much bone integration in vivo as titanium plasma spraying. One advantage of plasma coating is that it creates porous surface on implants with which bone may pierce them more easily. The thickness of less than 20 µm.[46]

Thermal Spraying

With its low cost and high deposition rate, thermal spraying HAP in implant devices is comparable to plasma spray coating. Depending on coating conditions, it can create a HA layer that ranges in thickness from 30 to 200 mm. Nevertheless, poor substrate adhesion and uneven crystallinity of films formed by thermal spraying shorten the lifespan of implants.

Thickness of 30-200 µm.[47] Sputtering process is particularly important procedure for deposition of Bioceramic thin films (based on Calcium/Phosphorous system), because of its capability to improved adhesion between coating and substrate ,providing greater control of its properties. Disadvantages are extensively time-taking, producing amorphous coatings & the Calcium/Phosphorous ratio coating is greater with that synthetic Hydroxyapatite. Thickness of 05-3 µm.

Magnetron sputtering

A viable thin-film technique that allows mechanical properties of Ti for preserving while maintaining bioactivity of coated Hydroxyapatite.[48]

Pulsed laser deposition

The method includes vaporizing bulk coating material from target using a high-power laser. Ejected from target, vaporized material condenses on substrate. A thin layer will deposit coating on the substrate as a outcome of repeated laser pulses.[49] Hydroxyapatite films produced by this method have low deposition temperatures and are highly crystalline, stable, osteoinductive. Thickness of 0.0S-5 mm.[50]

Dip Coating

By removing a substrate from liquid coating medium, wet liquid layer is deposited. The film's whole production process consists of many stages. On metal surfaces, HA may be uniformly coated to provide coating thickness between 0.05 and 0.5 mm. Without breaking down or reacting with the metal substrate, coating layer is applied to substrate's surface. Nevertheless, this method necessitates high sintering post treatments, which might cause cracks to appear on the substrate's surface.[51]

Sol-gel

In sol-gel, solid materials are formed from solution, mostly inorganic non-metallic compounds. Precursors that are oligomeric, monomeric, polymeric, or colloidal may be present in this solution. Since the sol-gel process operates at low temperatures, it is not affected by the structural instability of hydroxyapatite at high temperatures. Thickness of 0.1-2.0 μm.[52]

Electrophoretic deposition

It is a procedure whereby an electrode is coated with suspension particles while an electric field is present. Problems with the production of amorphous phases can be avoided by processing Hydroxyapatite electrophoretically at room temperature or below. Thickness of 0.1 -2.0 mm.[53]

Hot isostatic pressuring

An alternate technique for creating an HA coating on a Ti substrate is called hot isostatic pressing, in which the necessary Joad is exerted at desired temperature using compressed gas. For this, the porous HA-coated implant has to be encapsulated in a glass or metal that is gastight. Temperature & pressure are applied to workpiece simultaneously in the HIP process. Thickness of 0.2-2.0 mm.[54]

Ion Beam-assisted deposition

A vacuum deposition technique which combines physical vapor

deposition with ion beam bombardment. The use of this during deposition was the primary feature of ion beam-assisted deposition. Encouraging ions bombardment during deposition can help produce a large atomic intermixed zone between the substrate and coated material. As a result, coating adheres to the substrate strongly. Thickness is less than 0.03 μm.[5]

Photo functionalization

Ultraviolet light procedure of implant surfaces enhances osseointegration or bioactivity while altering titanium dioxide on surface. While inducing interactions of proteins & cell with implant on molecular level, UV light believed for enhancing osteoconductivity.[56]

Fluoride Treated

Depending on histomorphometric and biomechanical data, fluoride-modified titanium implants demonstrated firmer bone anchorage than unmodified, after short healing period. Formation of fluoridated Hydroxyapatite or fluorapatite with calcified tissues has been shown. Fluoride alteration has been linked to enhanced apatite crystal seeding rate, osteoprogenitor cell stimulation, elevated alkaline phosphatase activity, and integration of recently discovered collagen into bone matrix.[57]

Nanoparticle Compaction

Compaction of nanoparticles on implant surface conserves chemistry of underlying surface by modifying & replacing structure of outer surface layer.[58]

Peptide Coating

It involves coating of titanium Implant surface with synthetic arginyl-glycyl-aspartic acid peptides which comprise binding sites for integrin receptors.[59]

Antibiotic Coating

Antibiotics like amoxicillin, carbenicillin, cephalothin, cefamandole, gentamicin, vancomycin & tobramycin may bind with calcium-based coatings of implants, & released them which also retains its antimicrobial properties.[60]

Growth Factor Coating

Implant surface coated with osteogenesis-stimulating agents for accelerating bone formation or angiogenesis around it. Bone morphogenetic proteins (BMPs), vascular endothelial growth factors (VEGFs), transforming growth factor b1 (TGF-b1), insulin-like growth factors (IGFs) and platelet-derived growth factors (PDGFs), are some examples of these growth factors covering implants BMPs can be directly integrated in surface or using a plasmid that has gene which encodes BMPs.[61]

Bone Modulating Agent Coating

By using a biomimetic coating technique, implants can be coated with drugs linked to bone remodeling, such as bisphosphonates, which have strong chemical affinity for calcium phosphate molecules. Moreover, it may chemically incorporate into titanium in combination with RGD peptides to create synergistic osteogenic effects.[62]

SLA Treated

Roughening an implant's surface at the microscale has been conventional method of surface modification. Sandblasted, grit, and acid-etched (SLA) surfaces are among most effective surfaces in clinical dentistry. They are created by acid-etching a blasted surface and sandblasting it with large-grit particles, which typically have diameters between 250 and 500 μm. Strong acids including sulfuric, hydrochloric, and nitric acids are typically used for etching.[63] The treated material has an average surface roughness (Ra) of 1.5 pm.[64]

Chitosan Coating

It inhibited the development of P. gingivalis bacteria while permitting human gingival fibroblast cells to adhere and proliferate. It also demonstrated a high degree of cytocompatibility.[65]

White Surface Coating

Obtained using anodic plasma electrochemical oxidation of white-coated Ti topographies. It increases the production of osteocalcin and bone sialoprotein and has a beneficial effect on osteoblast cells, which proliferate quickly and promise an aesthetic appearance.[66]

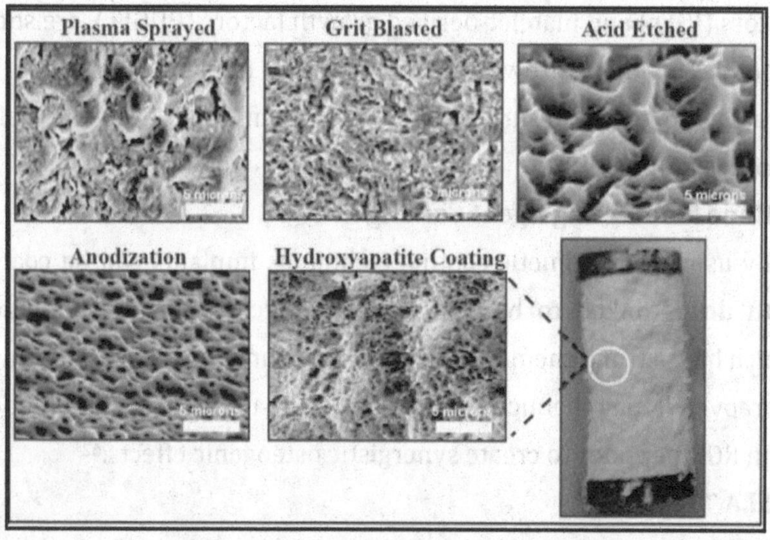

Fig.10 – Various surface treatment methods

4. STATE OF THE HOST BED

A key component of implant dentistry, available bone characterizes volume of the edentulous region and its exterior architecture. The density and quality of bone's interior are characterized, and these attributes reflect numerous biomechanical characteristics, including strength & elastic modulus. Internal or exterior bone architecture governs almost all aspects of implant dental practice. The amount of accessible bone in an edentulous location influences several aspects of prosthetic repair, including implant design, treatment planning, surgical technique, healing period, and initial progressive bone loading. [67,68]

Influence of Bone Density on Implant Success Rates

Arch location typically determines quality of bone.[67] Least dense bone is usually seen in posterior maxilla, while densest one anterior mandible, followed by posterior mandible. **Adell et al.**[69] claimed almost 10% higher success rate with anterior mandible compared to maxilla, using conventional surgical and prosthetic technique. When the same methodology was followed, **Schnitman et al.**[70] likewise observed reduced success rates in posterior mandible opposed with anterior. Posterior maxilla, which has lower bone density & larger force magnitude, has been shown to have highest reported clinical failure rates. As a result, there is an abundance of information on implant survival with regard for arch position.

In addition to arch location, several independent groups have reported different failure rates related with quality of bone.

According to **Engquist et al.**[71], soft bone types accounted for 78% of all reported implant failures. **Friberg et al.**[72] concluded that resorbed maxilla with soft bone accounted for 66% of their group's implant failures. A 5-year research, **Jaffin and Berman**[73] found that when low-density bone was seen in maxilla, there was a 44% implant failure rate. An article showed that in cases of low bone density, 35% of implants were lost in any part of the mouth. Soft bone types accounted for 55% of all implant failures in the research group.

According to **Johns et al.**[74], implants fail at a rate of 3% in moderate bone densities but at a rate of 28% in the weakest kind of bone. According to **Smedberg et al.**, 36% of patients with the lowest bone density failed.[75] The position of the arch has less of an impact on implant survival than bone density. **Snauwaert et al.**[76] discovered that maxilla was more likely to have early yearly and late failures in a follow-up analysis spanning 15 years. These documented failures happen after prosthetic loading rather than as a result of surgical healing. As a result, over a long period of time, several independent clinical groups that adhered to a uniform surgical protocol proved the undeniable impact of bone density on clinical outcome.

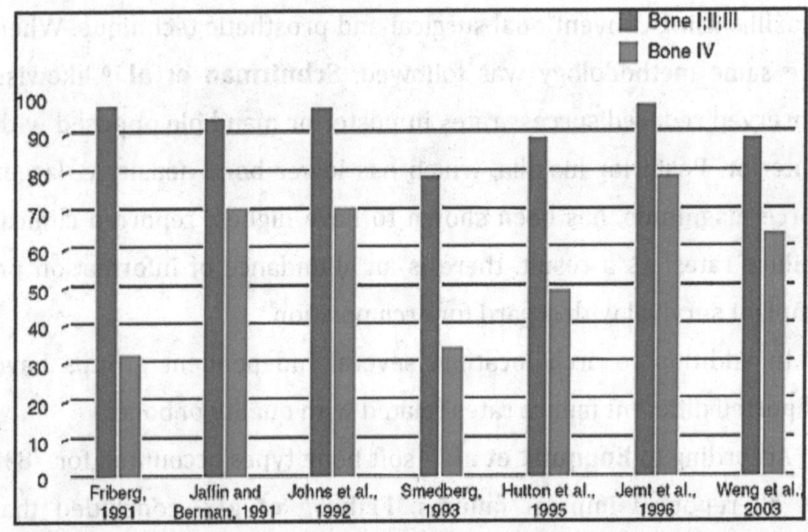

Fig.11 - Over the years, several clinical reports observed higher success rates in better bone quality and lower survival rates in poor bone quality (Bone IV).

Nevertheless, comparable success rates have been shown with all densities of bone & arch placements with a protocol developed by Misch—which modifies treatment strategy, selection of implant, surgical technique, regimen of healing, and first prosthetic loading—is followed.

5. SURGICAL CONSIDERATIONS

a. Optimal surgical technique to promote regenerative type rather than reparative bone healing.

b. Use of well-sharpened and graded series of drills.

c. Adequate cooling:- The critical time/temperature relationship for bone tissue necrosis is around 470 °C applied for one minute.

d. Slow drill speed (less than 2000 rpm and tapping at a speed of 15 rpm with irrigation).

e. A moderate power used at implant insertion

IMPACT OF DRILLING SPEED IN THE SUCCESS RATE OF IMPLANTOLOGY[77]

Endo-osseous implants in oral rehabilitation seem to safe & sensible option for successful treatment plan, success of those mostly based on how quickly bone healing progresses.[77] A thorough preparation of the site, which includes taking numerous precautions to minimize overheating following wear during osteotomy, is thought to be one of the key requirements for good healing among the many aspects affecting implant longevity. Heat generated during recipient site osteotomy causes necrosis, hyperemia, necrosis, osteocytic degeneration, fibrosis, and ultimately increasing osteoclastic activity, which degrades bone tissue and affects osseointegration, a crucial component of this kind of therapy.

The use of rotary drills or burs, which are necessary for site preparation, is frequently linked to bone necrosis brought on by heat and mechanical stress. The rotational osteotomy generates frictional heat, which causes an intrabony temperature shift. This overheating and subsequent heat transfer to bone is harmful to osseointegration & success rate of implant rehabilitation.

For the majority of implant systems with irrigation, high-speed drilling (between 800 and 1500 rpm) is advised in order to minimize bone overheating, maintain cell viability, avoid thermal necrosis, and shorten the time needed for osteotomy. Because of the low speed, longer drilling times are required, which increases the risk of heat generation from friction and scorching implant site.

Recent research, however, has returned the attention to low-speed drilling due to several potential advantages.[77] Crucial to remember that "drilling Speed" is just a several variables which might affect heat production, in turn, osseointegration, primary stability, bone vitality and maybe even size of particles in extracting bone for implant placement.

Operator	***Manufacturer***	***Site***	***Patient***
Drilling pressure	Drill design	Cortical thickness	Age
Drilling status	Irrigation system	Site condition	Bone density
Drilling motions	Drill sharpness	Drilling depth	
Drilling speed	Implant systems		
Drilling time			

1. **Drilling Speed and heat Generation:**

Sensitivity of bone to heat produced during bone drilling is perhaps most important factor which affect vitality and viability of bone at implant site & which requires to be taken into consideration. Success of endo-osseous implants is largely dependent on bone viability following implant site preparation. Many variables, including bone density, drilling depth, irrigation system, drill sharpness, load, feed rate, drilling wear etc., can cause heat generation during the bone drilling process.[77] Previous researches conducted by **Mathews & Hirsch**[78], **Rhinelander et al.**[79] on heat generation during implant osteotomy for evaluating critical bone temperature beyond that bone necrosis may occur had shown temperatures deleterious to bone tissue range from 56°C to 70°C as alkaline phosphatase is denatured at that level.[78,79]

Thompson conducted research on thermal changes & first histologic reactions for drilling bone at different speeds (125–2000 rpm) without the use of coolant. He found that as drilling speed increased, the temperature rose from 38.3°C to 65.5°C at 2.5 and 5 mm from the drill site.[80] As per treatment planning for osteotomy & reaming systems, a cooling system that combines both exterior & internal cooling may have superior option.[81]

In an analogous bone setting, **Matthews & Hirsch** investigated impact of temperature rise on drilling speed (345 -2900 rpm) and applied force (2 ,6, and 12 kg).[78] They came to the conclusion that, bone analogue, variations in drilling power were more likely to cause temperature to rise than other drilling parameters. Greater force reduces the production of heat. This was the first research to examine impact of load. In order to replicate the clinical circumstances associated with osteotomy, **Ji-Hyeon Oh et al.** observed heat generation during low-speed drilling process without irrigation in ten artificial bone blocks which simulated human D1 bone. Five fake bone blocks were drilled at 50 rpm without irrigation & five more in 1500 rpm with irrigation (control group). Thermocouples were utilized to detect the temperature shift. Drilling at moderate speed doesn't raise the temperature, as evidenced by the test group's average maximum change of 40.9ºC and control group's average maximum temperature change of 39.7ºC.[82]

Delgado-Ruiz et al. used a single-drill technique to study temperature changes in bone during implant osteotomy, but they controlled drill speed and design (50, 150, and 300 rpm) in artificial type IV bone.[83] The drill speed used by control group was 1200 rpm. Temperature rise with a single drill operation at a slow pace without irrigation, but it was still far below 47°C and determined that the sole factor influencing amount of time needed for an osteotomy in aforementioned case was drilling speed, with slower speeds requiring longer times.[83]

2. Drilling Speed, Bone Viability and Osseointegration

The bone type at implant osteotomy site and prevention of heat production are critical factors in effectiveness of osseointegration.[84,85] **Eduardo Anitua** investigated effect of low-speed drilling efficiency for viability & vitality of resulting particulate bone. He came to conclusion that crushed bone grafts may be useful in quick bone augmentation is required during a trial involving five patients.[86] "Live cells, maintained bone architecture, & significantly higher particle size" were seen in biologically drilled bone." **(Anitua, 2018, p.101)**

In 100 human subjects, **Tabrizi et al.** examined effects of drilling speeds (1000 rpm and 1500 rpm) and bone depth (10 mm & 13 mm) during implant osteotomy on bone viability. It was shown that while increasing depth or drilling speed alone does not affect mean percentage of bone cell vitality, doing so simultaneously can significantly lower proportion of viable bone.[87]

In their study, **Seo et al.** found that although higher provided better biological response, positive outcomes may be predicted with 50, 800, &1200 rpm drilling rates of mandible.[88]

3. Drilling Speed (DS) and Primary Stability (PS)

The primary stability during implant implantation is essential to long-term viability of dental implants. [88] It is related either to lack of mobility or bone integration. Primary stability is mostly determined by several factors, including implant thread design, surgical technique, and bone density and strength.

In a study conducted in vitro, **Georgios E. Romanos & colleagues** investigated the effects of "Drilling speed on PS of narrow diameter implants with different thread designs placed in dense and soft stimulated bone" **(Romanos 2004, p. 1350).** They found , for improved initial stability, a low drilling speed (800 rpm) is better in dense artificially stimulated bone than a high drilling speed (1200 rpm) in soft artificially simulated bone.[89]

In their sheep-based experimental animal study, **Ozcan et al.** compared the effects of four distinct osteotomy drilling speeds—50 rpm without saline cooling and 400 rpm, 800 rpm, 1200 rpm, and 2000 rpm with saline cooling—on temperature of cortical bone, implant stability, and bone healing. The temperature of cortical bone, primary and biological implant stability, and bone and tissue volume were found to be unaffected by drill speed during implant osteotomy & its irrigation. Nonetheless, a protracted preparation period with maximum primary stability, a high cortical bone temperature, and a drill speed of 50 rpm were observed.[90]

4. Drilling Speed and Particle Size

Studies assessing effect of drilling speed on size of recovered bone particles are few. **Chang-hee Jeong & colleagues** assessed how implant drilling speed affected composition of bone fragments extracted during drilling in a cow's jaw. A higher percentage of big particles were created by low-speed drilling.[91]

Tabassum et al. studied 20 patients utilizing low-speed drilling (200 rpm) without saline irrigation and normal drilling technique with saline irrigation.91 Better outcomes were obtained from autogenous bone particles extracted from low-speed drilling samples due to their osteogenic activity.[92]

BIOLOGICAL CONSIDERATIONS

INDICATIONS[93,94]

1. Retained Deciduous teeth

In cases where a permanent tooth is missing from birth, but deciduous teeth remain, an immediately placed implant can often be a viable solution.[95] Typically, a second premolar may be absent in either upper or lower jaw along with the deciduous baby molar. Early identification of these situations enables orthodontic development to achieve the optimal spacing between teeth before extraction. As long as anatomical structures like sinus and alveolar nerve are not at risk, deciduous teeth may be replaced by an implant after jaw has ceased growing.

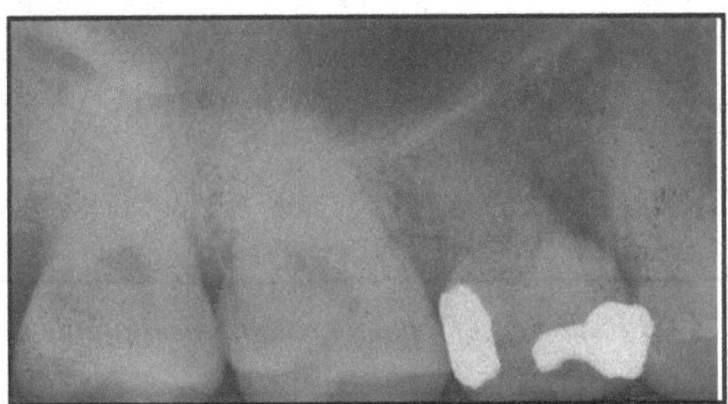

Fig.12 - Radiograph showing retained deciduous tooth E.

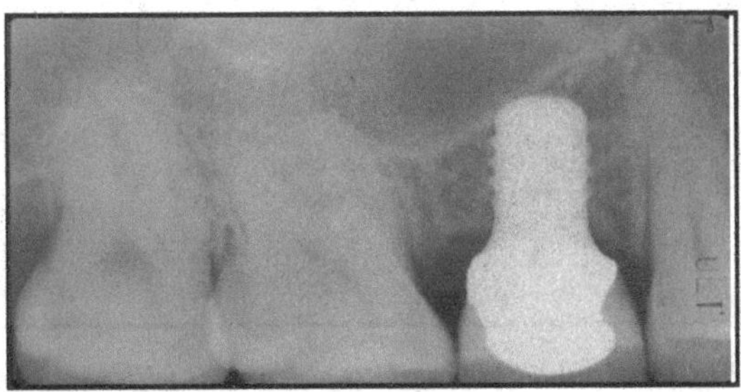

Fig.13 - Radiograph showing immediate implant replacing deciduous tooth E.

2. Non-restorable carious teeth

When dealing with a tooth that has severe subgingival caries, extracting it can present a chance for the surgeon to save crestal bone and associated gingival tissues while simultaneously placing an immediate implant. Typically, achieving primary stability in locations never challenging as surrounding alveolus remains undisturbed. Opting for immediate placement technique in such situations can also prove to be a cost-effective solution for the patient as opposed to other treatment options, which may require periodontics, restorative dentistry, endodontics, or orthodontics.

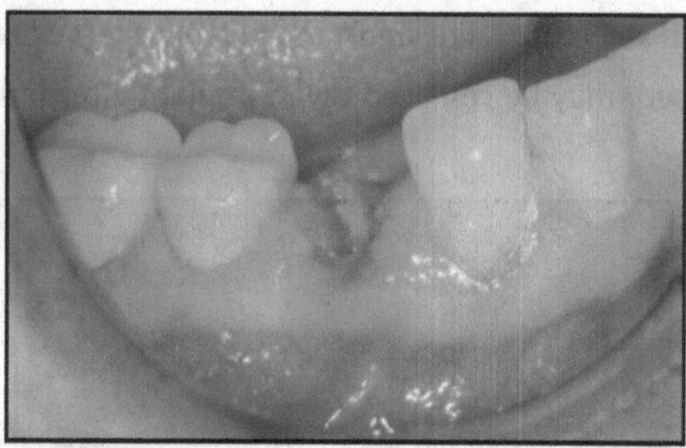

Fig.14 - Buccal view of tooth 44 with non-restorable caries

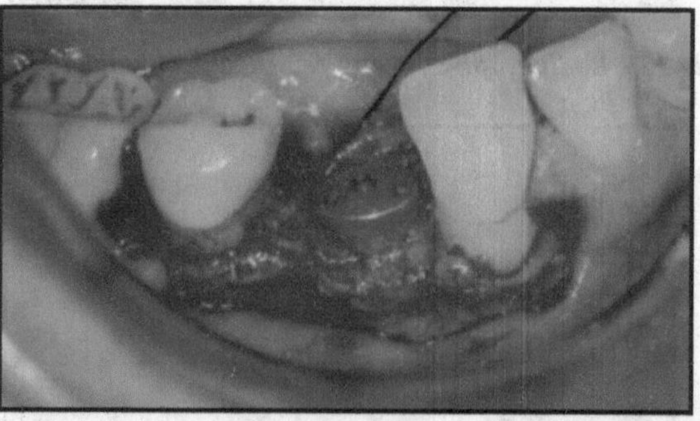

Fig.15 - Immediate implant placement with tooth 44

3. Vertical/Horizontal Root Fractures

Teeth that have been fractured at the root can be good candidates for immediate implant placement, provided that implant positioned ideally or there is primary stability.[96] However, if the fracture has been present for many week, there may be osseous defect that appears wide and narrow dehiscence. If these defect is present after implant placement, it may be corrected by using resorbable membrane or osseous graft prior to closing the flap.

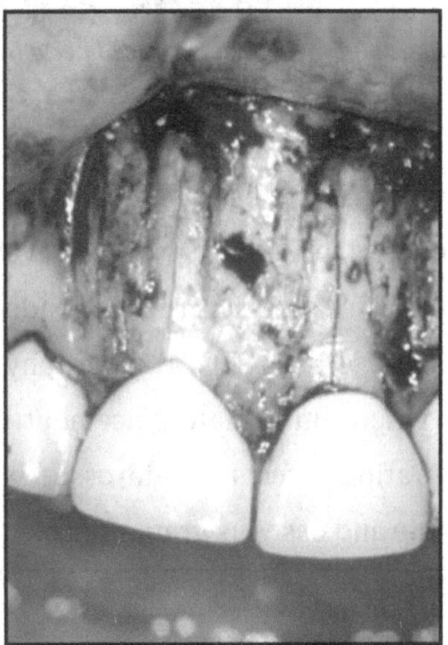

Fig.16 - Vertical Root Fractures

4. Periodontally Involved Teeth

Patients may experience advanced or refractory periodontal disease, which can result in tooth loss. Even with treatment, tooth loss may be unavoidable. In such cases, it was recommended for advising patient who have affected teeth or tooth extracted while there is sufficient alveolar bone for implant placement.[97]

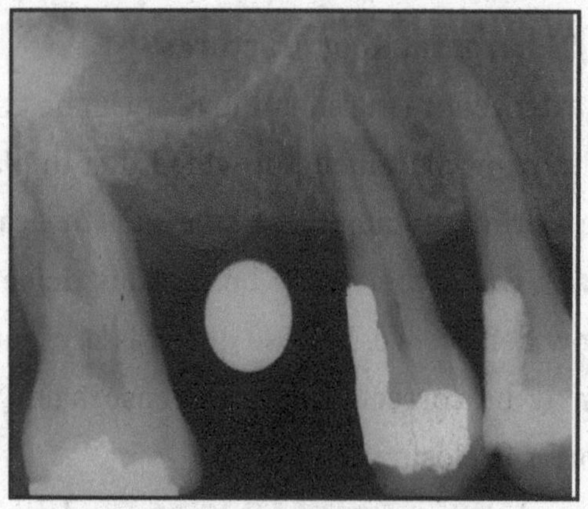

Fig.17 - Radiograph of teeth with reduced periodontal support.

5. Fenestration Defects

Research has found that opting for a flapless approach to implant placement may often lead to the buccal plates developing fenestration defects.[98] To prevent such issues, it is recommended to employ guided surgery procedures that utilizes CBCT radiography and surgical guide, especially in cases where immediate placement is planned.[99] When encountered, fenestration defects be addressed with combination of resorbable membrane and osseous graft after placing implant.[100]

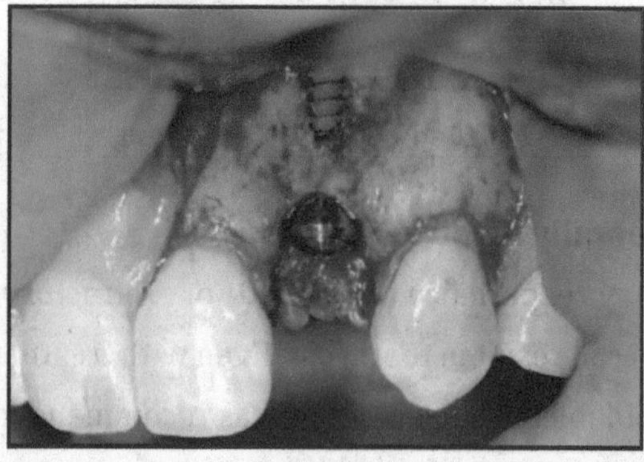

Fig.18 - fenestration defect following implant placement for tooth 26

CONTRAINDICATIONS [93,94]

1. Proximity to vital anatomic structures

Inferior Alveolar Nerve

While placing an immediate implant in posterior mandible, it is crucial accurately locate position of mental foramen or inferior alveolar nerve through radiography. Several rules have been established to caution clinician for maintaining atleast a 2mm distance from inferior alveolar nerve during osteotomy, implant placement, whether it is an early or delayed placement.[101]

Maxillary Sinus

It can be challenging to place an immediate implant in second premolar, 1st &2nd molar sites due to position of maxillary sinus.[102] In some cases, 2nd premolar site may be too wide and 4.8 mm diameter implant may not provide enough stability by engaging lateral walls of socket. To address this issue, early placement protocol is recommended for reducing socket dimensions and ensure stability or predictability.

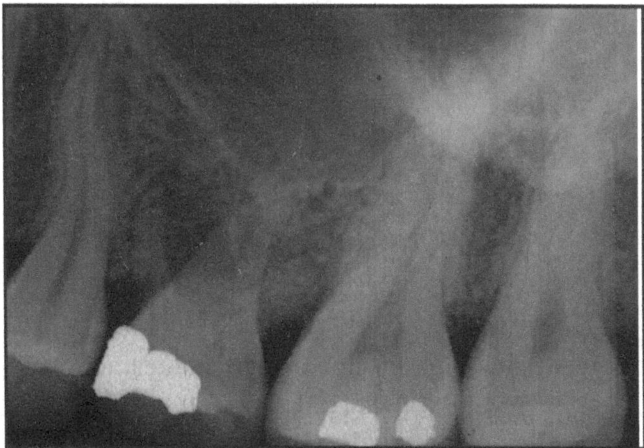

Fig.19 - Radiograph of deciduous tooth J and the proximity to the maxillary sinus floor

2. Sites requiring guided bone regeneration

Trauma and infection-affected areas may exhibit notable loss in lingual or buccal bone plate, exposing sizable portion of implant surface right away. While initial stability can be attained, guided bone regeneration (GBR) is preferred method for reconstructing alveolar ridge in order to maximize aesthetics and enhance outcomes, particularly for anterior area.[103]

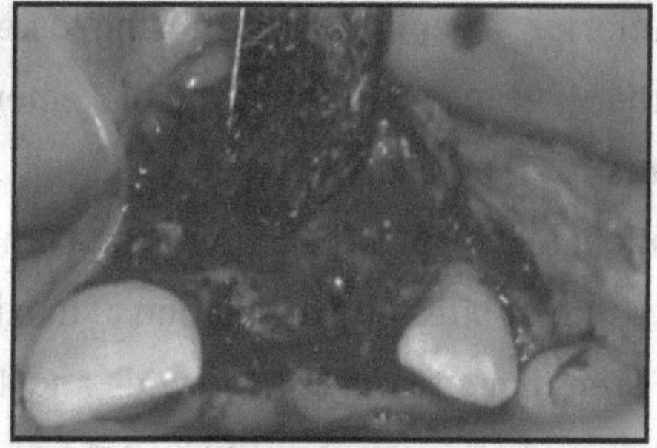

Fig.21 - Occlusal view of 22 following GBR.

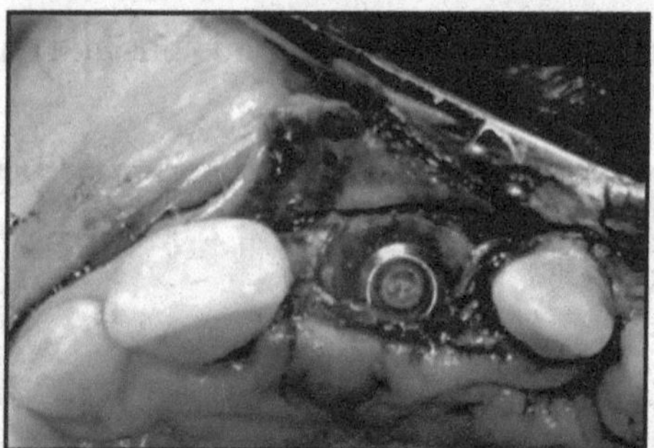

Fig.20 - Occlusal view of 22 requiring GBR.

3. Patients with high lip line

Patients who have high lip line and broad aesthetic area should informed about possibility for having final restoration which might not be symmetrical with the contra-lateral tooth.[1] It is recommended to avoid immediate placement in cases where there is a potential for marginal tissue recession that can't controlled in high smile line situation. A staged approach can give more predictable outcome in such situations.

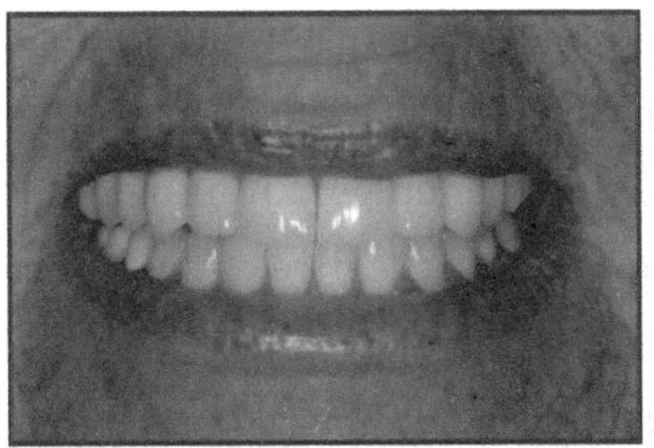

Fig.24 - High Smile Line

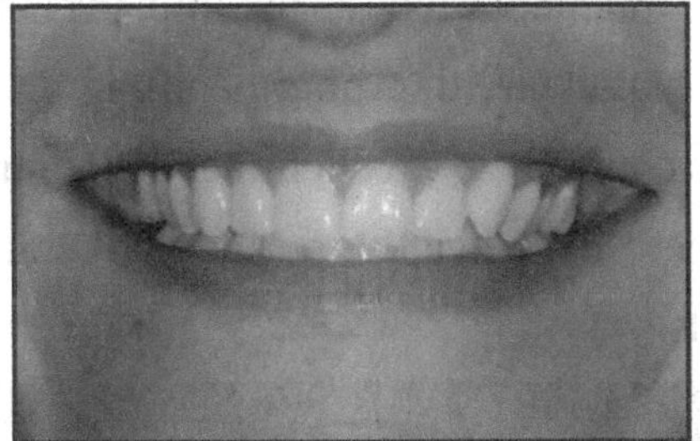

Fig.22 - Low Smile Line

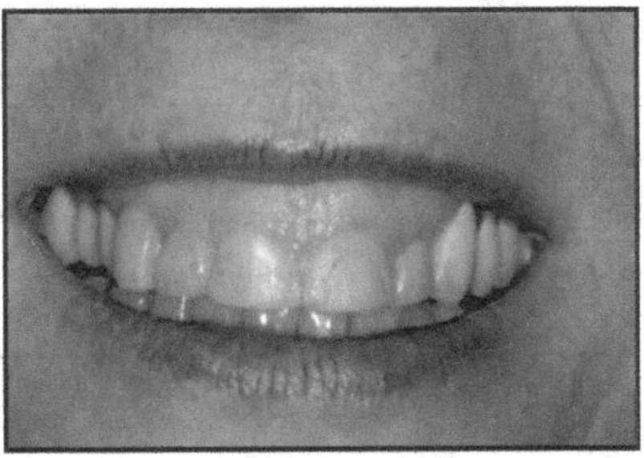

Fig.23 - Medium Smile Line

4. Tissue phenotype

Tissue phenotypes have specific visual and situational characteristics which can affect appearance or long-term stability of soft tissues surrounding implants. Most favorable phenotype for clinician for managing is thick tissue phenotype.[105] This type of tissue is more resistant to marginal tissue recession and can conceal metallic color of implant &associated restorative parts, particularly when implant is positioned at shallow dimension. However, it's important to note that thick tissue phenotype may be more susceptible in healing by scar formation when vertical releasing incisions necessary for assessing operating site.

Thin tissue phenotypes are not very common then too can pose certain challenges. In such cases, it is recommended to provide both hard & soft tissue augmentation during implant insertion & position implant slightly palatally. With proper handling, an implant with thin tissue phenotype could have excellent aesthetic outcome, especially when adjacent teeth have healthy periodontal status and unaltered crestal bone levels.[105]

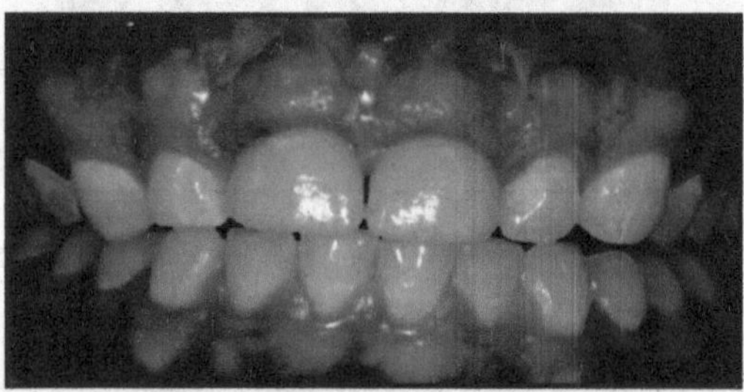

Fig.25 - Thick Gingival Phenotype

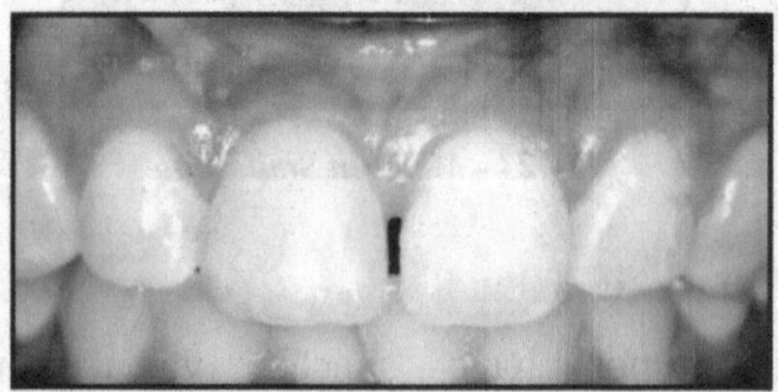

Fig.26 - Thin Gingival Phenotype

Dehiscence defects

It is often noticed that thin buccal bone crests associated with dehiscence before extracting teeth and frequently develop iatrogenically during extraction, even with most experienced and careful clinician.[106] Although occurrence and observation of buccal dehiscence should not necessarily prevent proceeding with immediate placement technique, it does require clinician to reconstruct the defect us osseous graft with low substitution rate. Additionally, bioresorbable membranes should be applied at time of implant placement to aid in repair process.[107]

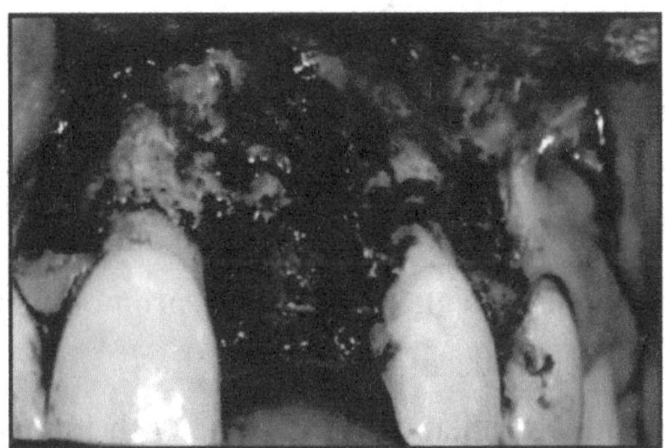

Fig.27 - Long Dehiscence defect involving tooth 21.

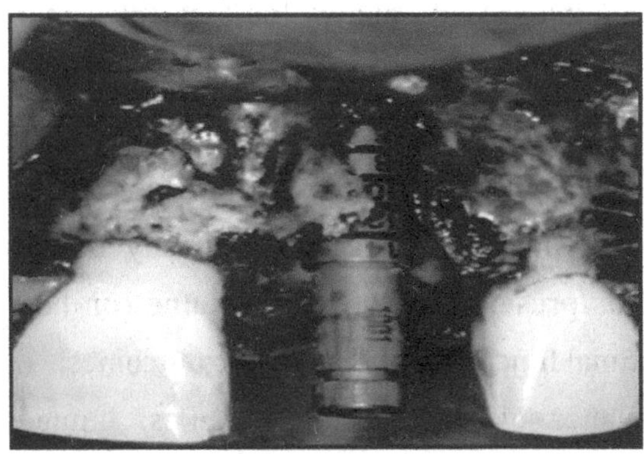

Fig.28 - Depth Gauge in Place During the Treatment of Tooth 21 With an Immediate Implant.

THE ADVANTAGES OF IMMEDIATE IMPLANT PLACEMENT INCLUDE:[4]

1. Reduce in a number of surgical interventions: Immediate implant placement allows for combining tooth extraction & implant placement in a single surgical procedure. This eliminates the need for a separate surgery for implant placement, reducing overall surgical interventions.
2. Reduced treatment duration: By placing implant immediately after tooth extraction, treatment duration is significantly reduced while comparing to delayed implant placement. This can lead to faster restoration of the missing tooth or teeth.
3. Preservation of alveolar bone width and height: Immediate implant placement helps preserve alveolar bone, which is bone surrounding socket. This preservation allows for maximum utilization of the bone-implant surface area, promoting better implant stability and long-term success.
4. Achieving ideal implant orientation: With immediate implant placement, it can be positioned optimally in terms of angulation, depth, and alignment. This allows for ideal placement of implant relative to adjacent teeth and overall dental arch.
5. Preservation of bone at extraction site: Immediate implant placement helps maintain bone in extraction site while preventing or minimizing resorption of bone that typically occurs after tooth extraction. This preservation of bone volume can be beneficial for achieving optimal functional and aesthetic outcomes.
6. Maintenance of soft tissue aesthetics: Immediate implant placement can help preserve the gingival contour and architecture, contributing for better soft tissue aesthetics around implant

restoration. This can result in a more natural-looking smile.

7. Improved patient acceptance: Immediate implant placement offers few advantage with respect to reduced treatment duration, preservation of bone, soft tissue, and better aesthetic outcomes. These factors contribute to improved patient acceptance and satisfaction with the overall implant treatment.

THE DISADVANTAGES OF IMMEDIATE IMPLANT PLACEMENT INCLUDE:[108]

1. Risk of partial alveolar bone resorption: There is a potential risk of partial bone resorption at the implant site, especially if there is an underlying pathological process or if there is traumatic damage to the alveolar bone during the tooth extraction. This can affect stability and long-term success of implant.
2. Difficulty while achieving primary stability: Immediate implant placement may be more challenging to achieve optimal primary stability compared to delayed implant placement. Immediate placement relies on the existing bone structure without the opportunity for pre-implant site preparation or bone healing.
3. Gap between implant surface and socket wall: When placing it immediately after extraction, there can be space between socket wall and implant surface. This can hinder proper bone-to-implant contact & osseointegration, potentially affecting long-term success of implant.
4. Additional cost for GBR: In cases of inadequate bone volume for IIP, guided bone regeneration procedure can be needed to augment bone. This can increase overall cost of treatment.
5. Difficulty in predicting final position of implant: Immediate implant placement presents challenges in accurately predicting final position of implant because of few factors such as socket morphology

and tissue response. This can impact functional and aesthetic outcomes of implant restoration.

6. Difficulty in achieving complete closure of the implant site: Achieving complete closure of soft tissue at implant site might be challenging with immediate implant placement. This can increase risk of complications like delayed healing & infection

7. Need for flap elevation in two-stage procedures: In cases where a two-stage implant placement approach is preferred, which involves placing the implant below the gumline and covering it with a flap, there is a need to raise a flap for proper implant coverage. This adds a surgical step and can potentially lead to increased discomfort and prolonged healing.

RATIONALES FOR IMMEDIATE IMPLANT PLACEMENT.[93]

1. **Predictable Outcome**:

IIP offers predictable results in terms of osseointegration or long-term success. It allows for better preservation of alveolar bone and soft tissue contours.

2. **High Acceptance and Patient Satisfaction:**

Patients often prefer immediate implant placement due to reduced treatment time and fewer surgical procedures. The ability to restore function and aesthetics promptly contributes to higher patient satisfaction.

3. **One Surgery vs. Two or Three Procedures:**

Immediate implant placement combines implant placement and tooth extraction into a single surgical procedure. This reduces overall number of surgeries and simplifies treatment process.

4. **Fixed Temporary Restoration:**

When indicated, a provisional bridge or crown can be immediately placed on implant. This provides functional and aesthetic benefits during healing period and enhances patient comfort.

5. Fewer Scheduled Appointments:

Immediate implant placement streamlines the treatment timeline, requiring fewer follow-up appointments. Patients appreciate the convenience and efficiency.

6. Less Time Elapsed Before Final Restoration:

Typically, the final restoration (such as a permanent crown) can be placed within 3–4 months after immediate implant placement. This shorter waiting period benefits both patients and clinicians.

KEY ELEMENTS IN IMMEDIATE IMPLANT PLACEMENT SURGERY[109]

1. Use caution when starting with a pilot drill since there is a chance of it sliding into socket and puncturing buccal bone plate due to hardness of palatal wall. In order of circumventing issue, 2 methods have been suggested:

a) When implantation occurs immediately with little or very little tissue loss, round bur method is recommended. A little circular bur that is roughly one-third of apex on palatal wall of socket is used to start the drilling process. After that, drilling is done while maintaining palatal orientation concerning tooth axis. If residual area more than 2 mm, bone cannot be recovered and must be filled by a grafting substance

b) The trepan process improves axis implant control while allowing bone to regenerate for further filling. In order to maximize main stability of implant, drilling should be done beyond socket during implant site preparation. Drilling done beyond an apical lesion for eliminating contaminated tissue and provide a stable anchoring in healthy tissue.

2. Choice of an implant of an adequate diameter as per anatomical and prosthetic requirements. Complete inter-dental papilla fill is substantially correlated with 3–4 mm horizontal gap with neighbouring implants/teeth & 3–5 mm vertical in between contact point or inter-proximal bone. Seldom does the implant axis align with the socket axis:-

a) At upper-anterior region, implant is placed more palatal than extraction socket, for upper molars and premolars with 2 roots, it is placed at level of septum.

b) At lower molar region, implant is placed at inter-radicular septum.

c) For lower-anterior region, implants are as parallel as possible.

REVIEW OF LITERATURE

1. **Meijer HJA, Raghoebar GM (2020)**[110] conducted a study involving fifteen patients with single failing molar of upper and lower jaw, who underwent implant treatment with 2-staged surgical technique. 3 months later, full contour screw-retained zirconia restoration was provided. Radiographic & clinical examinations performed one-twelve months after restoration. Results showed a 73.3% implant and restoration survival rate at one-year evaluation, to mean marginal bone loss of 0.17 mm. While limitations existed, research demonstrated a high implant failure rate with immediate placement of regular diameter implants in molar post-extraction sites at mandible and maxilla.

2. **Slagter KW, Raghoebar GM, Hentenaar DFM, Vissink A, Meijer HJA (2021)**[111] Their Goal of study was to evaluate, in aesthetic region after 5 years of function, changes in marginal bone level around immediately put & professionalized implants with those installed and delayed provisionalized implants. Forty patients of maxillary front area who had a failing tooth were randomly allocated for either a delayed (Group B: n = 20) /immediate implant insertion with immediate provisionalization (Group A: n = 20). Mean changes in distal and mesial marginal bone levels after five years didn't determine significant difference between both groups (p =.477 and.305, respectively). There were no clinically significant variations in buccal bone thickness & mid-facial peri-implant mucosal level, aesthetics, and patient result. Survival rates of implants and restorations were 100%. Study found that average marginal changes in bone level after provisionalization and IIP were similar.

3. **Garcia-Sanchez R, Mardas N, Buti J, Ortiz Ruiz AJ, Pardo Zamora G (2021)**[112] compared the success and survival rates, Modified success rate, survival, buccal bone thickness, & patient-reported results of immediate dental implants employing flap or minimal split-thickness envelope flap (MSTEF) implanted in newly created alveolar sockets. There were no statistically significant variations seen in PES, WES scores (Pink and White Esthetic Scores), or success criteria including aesthetic factors across the 28 patients who had total of 28 implants. There were no statistically significant variations in buccal wall thickness or patient-reported outcomes, and survival rates were 100%. Similar mean PES/WES ratings, survival,mean buccal bone levels, modified success rate, & patient satisfaction were obtained with immediate dental implant therapy of flap/MSTEF; however, cosmetic failures were frequent in both groups.

4. **Crippa R, Aiuto R, Dioguardi M, Nieri M, Peñarrocha-Diago M, Peñarrocha-Diago M, et al. (2023)**[113]conducted a study between 2014 and 2019 that compared conventional implants of edentulous sites (control) to immediate post-extraction implants with infected sites treated with laser (test group). Study included a minimum one-year follow-up period and examined clinical history, pre- and postoperative radiographs. Only one (1%), out of the 149 implants under study, failed in test group; no failures occurred in control. In comparison baseline, test group increased their MBL by 0.1 mm, while control had a decrease in MBL of 0.1 mm. Two groups' mere 0.2 mm difference, however, did not reach statistical significance (P = 0.058). According to findings, dental implants placed right away in diseased sockets after they have been debrided or cleaned use an Er,Cr:YSGG

laser do not raise risk of failure. However, stringent guidelines and procedures are needed to prevent peri-implantitis and related issues.

5. **Hirani M, Moshtofar Z, Devine M, Paolinelis G, Djemal S (2023)**[114] evaluated efficacy of immediate implant placed to anterior maxilla following dental trauma. Study included 60 patients who were treated with 70 implants, resulting to an implant survival rate of 95.7% over 3 year follow-up period. Prosthetic survival was examined at 100%, in favourable periodontal outcomes. Study shown that IIP can be reliable treatment strategy. However, future well-designed clinical trials needed for examine long-term result of procedure.

6. **Çolak S, Demïrsoy MS (2023)**[115] conducted a study that examined 69 patients & 124 immediate implants within three groups. Success rates were 97.2% ,93.5%,81.8% in Group 1, 2,3 respectively. The $\chi 2$ test showed significant correlation between study groups & implant success rates ($p = 0.037$). Smoking was also found to have a significant relationship with implant success ($p = 0.015$). Immediate implant placement had high survival rates in sockets of periapical pathology, with satisfactory success rates to guided bone regeneration. However, simultaneous sinus lifting technique had significantly lower success rates. Adequate curettage and debridement in sockets with periapical pathology showed high implant survival rates. Future treatment protocols should progress in safer ways as complexity of surgical procedures increases.

7. **Bambini F, Memè L, Rossi R, Grassi A, Grego S, Mummolo S (2023)**[116] suggested a novel method for employing next-generation REX-type blade implants for immediate post-extraction implants. With this method, implants were placed into the septum right after extraction. At the 18-month follow-up, 20 patients' REX implants

were found stable & encircled with newly produced bone. Because this treatment facilitates periosteal inhibition, it allowed for high patient compliance & preservation of alveolus. Positive clinical outcomes indicated that even in situations including post-extraction sockets, this method can avoid surgical procedures. To fully grasp method's potential for use in routine clinical practice, more clinical research is needed.

8. **Bahaa A, Bahaa AM, El-Bagoury N, Khaled N, Ibrahim AM (2024)**[117] investigated whether dual-zone treatment idea might be used immediately for implant insertion in posterior extraction sockets. Five non-restorable molars or premolars were included in trial, and eleven implants were placed right away following a painless piezotome extraction. The dual-zone therapy approach included using a screw-retained, tailored healing abutment to promote healing after a bovine xenograft was used to fill jumping gap next to implant up to gingival margin. The patients were monitored for three years to evaluate peri-implant marginal tissue health, implant or prosthesis loss, and surgical complications. Implant loading was postponed for four to six months. During follow-up appointments, findings revealed no surgical problems or implant loss. Excellent outcomes were shown in peri-implant marginal tissue health, with little marginal bone loss and, in certain cases, visible bone growth. Long-term success in posterior extraction sockets seems to be possible with dual-zone treatment paradigm combined with rapid implant insertion.

PROTOCOLS FOR IMMEDIATE IMPLANT PLACEMENT

Immediate Implants in Aesthetic Zone

According to available data, gingival biotype, integrity and thickness of buccal bone plate are crucial elements which are in instantaneous implants' success. For papilla formation, a three mm gap between implants is ideal. For preventing soft tissue recession, a buccal plate with minimum of one mm and an average of 2 mm is ideal. The buccal position of implants will be avoided when adhering to immediate implant protocol. Implants ought to be positioned lingually or palatally. A gingival biotype that is thicker is preferable. High scalloping gingiva may raise the chance of a recession. The interproximal bone's location affects the soft tissue architecture as a whole.[118]

Piezosurgery or Periotomes can be used to extract teeth with the least amount of soft tissue trauma and mucoperiosteal flap. Self-tapping implants enhance primary stability that compresses alveolar bone as implant is inserted. Bone substitutes with a low rate of resorption should be used to fill space that exists between implant & interior surface of facial bone wall, which is 2 mm.[119] Implant is positioned at least 1 millimeter apical to buccal ridge and two - three millimeters from gingival margin to account for the anticipated vertical resorption.

Another crucial element is primary implant stability, which calls for either engaging bone apical for original socket dimensions or lateral walls without altering original depth. For immediate implant placement, tapered design implant will advantageous. Furthermore, a flapless surgical technique, use of platform switch implants, simultaneous implantation for CTG or use of temporary restorations right away could all be considered. Completion of IIP in aesthetic area necessitates highly skilled surgery, optimal extraction socket conditions, and local anatomy knowledge. Other implant duration protocols which produced good clinical results for both soft and hard tissues should be followed in absence to ideal conditions.[120]

Implant placement in aesthetic zone sites be avoided when using a wide platform or wide diameter. Implants with a diameter of roughly four mm are typically used to treat mandibular cuspids or premolars, as well as maxillary. Implant in the mandibular and lateral incisor regions shouldn't have a diameter larger than 3.5 mm.[94]

To summarize, clinical guidelines for immediate implant placement protocol are mentioned below:-

- Intact and thick buccal bone wall
- Thick gingival biotype
- Minimal trauma in tooth extraction
- Presence of at least three socket walls—ideally four walls
- Implant design
- Implant shoulder should be placed 2–3 mm apical to anticipated gingival margin
- Primary implant stability
- Slight lingual or palatal positioning of the implant
- Fill gap

Immediate Implants in the Posterior Region

Implant positioning of root socket may result in a less-than-ideal restorative position in the posterior region. This could lead to a mechanical overload and implant failure. With addition, resulting structure of restoration may render oral hygiene more difficult, that increases chances of periimplantitis.[118]

Studies have recommended implant placement into inter-radicular bone and membrane and graft material augmentation of the remaining socket to circumvent these possible issues.[93] Even though there isn't much information available in the literature regarding immediate molar implants' long-term performance, when used by qualified clinicians, it seems like a viable treatment option. Clinicians should adhere to stringent guidelines due to the intricacy of the procedure to reduce the likelihood of complications or failures.[118]

Clinical guidelines for immediate implant placement in posterior region –

- Patients should be non-smokers.
- A pre-operative CBCT scan for minimizing risk, mostly in mandible.
- Thick gingival biotype and adequate keratinized tissue width (≥ 2 mm).
- Atraumatic extraction with flap-less surgery if feasible.
- Only sites of intact socket walls after extraction.
- Osteotomy preparation will vary with socket type
- Implants to be submerged (up to 2 mm) below buccal bone crest if crestal buccal bone is thin (<2 mm).
- Thin buccal plate (<2 mm) may require more lingual placement implant with gap grafting or buccal over-grafting.
- Gaps between socket walls & implant are generally grafted if ≥ 2 mm in width.
- Xenograft and mineralized allograft preferred.
- Initial implant stability should be established.

- Submerged healing if primary stability is less than 25 and resonance frequency value less than 60.

OSSEOUS DENSIFICATION

Over the years, endosseous implants have proven to have success rates of over 90%, and one of the key components of that success is thought to be implant stability. Various factors are said to affect initial biomechanical primary stability, like osteotome and drilling surgical preparation procedure, bone mineral density,type & length,diameter, taper, surface design and threading parameters of implant.[121]

Direct, structural, & functional attachment of live bone for an implant surface known as osseointegration, and it thought to be mandatory condition for implant loading & long-term clinical success. Two parameters have significant impact with success of endosseous implants: direct microscopic implant-to-bone contact & amount and quality of histology bone structure at implant interface, that is significantly connected with bone mineral density. It has been demonstrated that preserving majority of bone mineral & collagen material together with enhanced primary stability might quicken healing process following surgery. To guarantee a successful endosseous implantation, it is crucial to retain bone's histologic structure & preserving bone mass in osteotomy preparation process.

Drilling is widely established procedure employed for preparing bone for implant placement. It involves surgical procedure of cutting and extracting bone tissue to create a cylindrical osteotomy, which is intended to receive an implant fixture. Designed to provide best possible bone cutting, twist drills usually have two or three flutes with rake angles between 25 and 35 degrees on the cutting blades. However, bone loss during drilling may jeopardize pullout strength and stability of implant fixation. If proper cooling and irrigation are not used, drilling may also result in additional clinical consequences such heat generation-induced osteonecrosis. Moreover, geometric precision of osteotomy may be adversely affected by drill-tip skiving over bone surface and vibration brought on by a continuously shifting cutting resistance vector as a result of non-uniform bone characteristics.

The **Osseous Densification technique**, developed by **Huwais**[122] in 2013, is a bone preservation method that utilizes specially designed bur with multiple lands and large negative rake angle. When these non-cutting edges enlarge an osteotomy, density of bone is increased. Bone is gently compacted by densifying burs, which having four or more lands and flutes. These are surgical instruments featuring a tapered shank and a cutting chisel edge. They have a steadily growing diameter which regulates expansion process as they go further into osteotomy. When using these burs, a typical surgical engine is utilized. By spinning in non-cutting direction (counter-clockwise at 800-1,200 rotations per minute) and cutting direction (clockwise at 800-1,200 rotations per minute), they may densify/ drill bone.

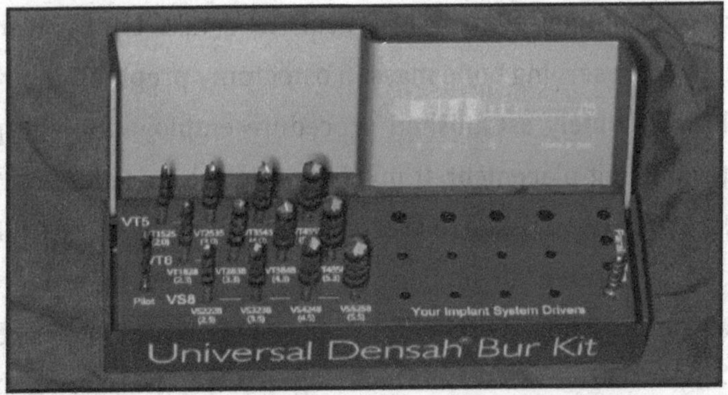

Fig.29 - Versah Kit with densification drills

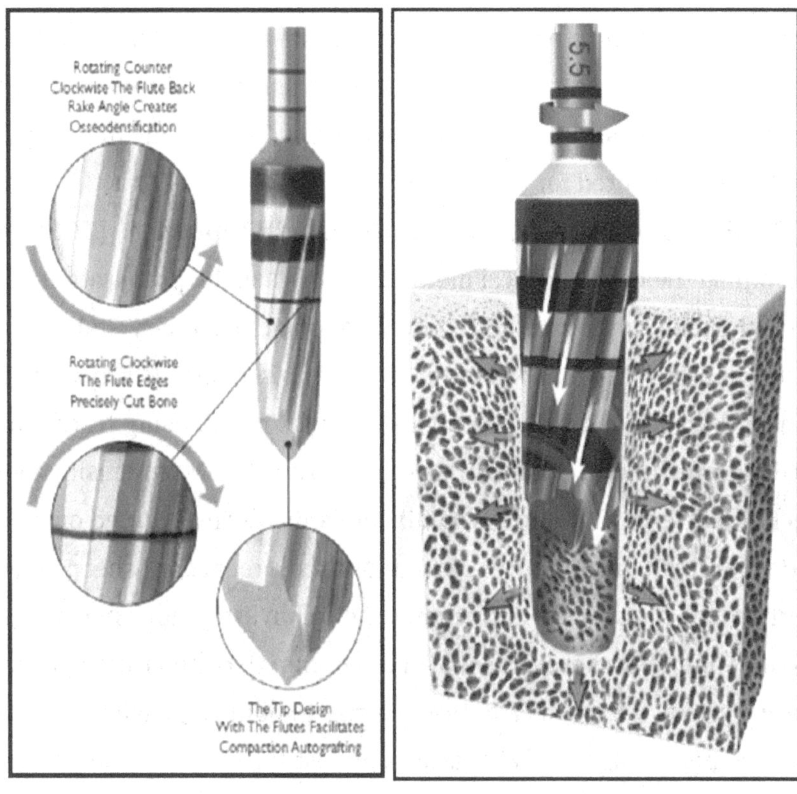

Figs.30 & 31 - Role of densification Drills

Compaction autografting is a dynamic, non-subtractive bone instrumentation technique used to increase bone density. By applying controlled deformation as a result of sliding or rolling contact for revolving lands of densifying bur along with inner surface of osteotomy, bone compaction is achieved. In this process, greater volumes of irrigation fluid are used for preventing overheating & to lubricate surfa of bur and bone. Prior to moment of contact, a pressure wave can be created by using bur to bounce in and out of osteotomy. The autografting of bone fragments along inner surface of osteotomy is aided by irrigation fluid that is pushed into it. For further densify inner walls and create a density crust along whole depth of osteotomy, compaction autografting using densifying drills complements basic bone compression effect. This results in a surface that is well-adapted for the implant.[123]

Trisi P, Berardini M, Falco A, Podaliri Vulpiani M (2016)[124] examined the novel surgical method for implant site preparation that would enable improved ridge width, implant secondary stability, & bone density. Ten 3.8 × 10-mm Dynamix implants (Cortex) were placed in left sides of 2 sheep-exposed iliac crests using traditional drilling technique (control). Using Versah Osseodensification technique, ten 5 × 10-mm Dynamix implants (Cortex) placed on right sides of test group. After two month of recovery, sheep were euthanized, histological and biomechanical investigations performed. No implant failures were seen over a two-month recuperation period. In test group, there was a noticeable rise in both ridge width & bone volume percentage (%BV) that was almost thirty percentile greater. While comparing to control, test group showed much improved removal torque values and micromotion under lateral stresses. Compared to traditional implant drilling procedures, Osseodensification approach utilized in-vivo study was shown to be able to improve percentage BV surrounding dental implants put in low-density bone. This contributed in improving stability and decreasing micromotion.

Ibrahim A., Ayad S., ElAshwah A. (2020)[125] assessed Osseodensification (OD) procedure efficacy at implant site preparation with recently developed Densah bur. Ten individuals had twenty dental implants put. In posterior maxillary ridge, each patient got one implant drilled using Osseodensification approach and one drilled using conventional technique. Osstell was used to test implants' stability by determining their resonance frequency (ISQ-scale). Using Densah bursts significantly improved both primary and secondary stability, as per data. Compared to traditional drills, this improved quality of bone surrounding implant, enhancing both primary and secondary stability.

Bergamo ETP, Zahoui A, Barrera RB, Huwais S, Coelho PG, Karateew ED, et al. (2021)[126] in a multicenter clinical trial, gave 56 patients a total of 150 implants and were assessed using regular, narrow, and wide implants, as well as regular, short, and long implants in specific regions of maxilla and mandible. Osteotomies were performed following manufacturer recommendations. The results showed that Osseodensification (OD) yielded higher IT (Insertion Torque) and ISQ (Implant Stability Quotient) value compared with Subtractive Drilling (SD) across various parameters, except for small implants. Overall, OD shown superior performance relative to SD in terms of ISQ and IT values, independent to healing time and specific implant dimensions and locations.

Stacchi C, Troiano G, Montaruli G, Mozzati M, Lamazza L, Antonelli A, et al. (2023)[127] compared the stability of implant changes during first 90 days healing after using Osseodensification (OD) or Piezoelectric implant site preparation (PISP). Total 27 patients received two identical implants in posterior maxilla, with one site prepared using OD and the other using Piezoelectric site preparation. Resonance frequency analysis performed at different intervals, and after one year loading, 53 out of 54 implant functioning well. The study observed no significant differences in stability of implant or survival rate between two preparation methods.

Costa JA, Mendes JM, Salazar F, Pacheco JJ, Rompante P, Moreira JF, et al. (2024)[128] examined variations in bone density and contrasted implant placement techniques using Osseodensification and traditional osteotomy. A total of 41 implants were placed in 15 patients—20 for traditional osteotomy, 21 through osseodensification. One year following prosthetic rehabilitation, a cone beam computed tomography carried out to evaluate bone density. Median density values of 1020 following osseodensification were substantially greater than those of 732 with traditional bone drilling, according to the results. It was determined that no statistically significant correlation with sex, implant size, site area, main implant stability and bone density in either approach. The study found that over a year, osteodensification enhanced bone density.

CLINICAL REQUIREMENTS TO BE FULFILLED FOR ATTAINING HIGH SUCCESS RATES FOR IMMEDIATE IMPLANT PLACEMENT (IIP)[129]

1. **Absence of Active Infection:**

a. Active infections can compromise healing and implant integration.

b. Address any existing infections through appropriate treatment (such as root canal therapy or extraction) before proceeding with IIP.

2. **Mechanical Anchorage and Stability:**

a. The implant fixture must achieve good primary stability within the alveolar socket.

b. Adequate bone density and quality are crucial for achieving this stability.

c. Proper implant site preparation and precise placement contribute to mechanical anchorage.

3. **Atraumatic Tooth Removal:**

a. The unsalvageable tooth should be extracted gently and atraumatically.

b. Minimize trauma of surrounding soft tissue and bone in extraction.

c. Preservation of alveolar bone is essential for successful implant placement.

4. **Labial Plate Preservation:**

a. The labial (front) plate of bone should be preserved during tooth extraction.

b. This ensures adequate bone support for implant and maintains esthetics.

c. Ridge augmentation or socket preservation may help in maintaining bone volume.

5. Appropriate Implant Design:

a. Choose an implant design that matches the socket's configuration.

b. Consider factors such as implant diameter, length, and thread design.

c. Customized abutments may be necessary to achieve optimal emergence profile.

6. Precise Implant Positioning:

a. Implant angulation and position play a critical role in long-term success.

b. Proper alignment with adjacent teeth and occlusion is essential.

c. Use surgical guides or navigation systems to achieve accurate implant placement.

SURGICAL INSTRUMENTATION[130]

Surgical instrumentation kits include an assortment of ***drills, drivers, wrenches, screw taps,*** and ***implant mounts.***

Implant Drills

Osteotomies are made in bone using implant drills, which are rotating cutting tools. They are constructed from a variety of material, like ceramics, surgical stainless steel and titanium alloy. Drills are made to produce right osteotomy size and shape when used in right order with suggested torque, irrigation, and rotary speed. This provides initial stability without putting the bone through mechanical or thermal stress.

Drivers

Various drivers are included in the surgical kit, depending on the manufacturer. Screws used in the course of implant treatment are engaged with hexed, slotted, or unigrip drivers.

Implant Mounts

Some systems require an implant mount to be attached to the implant to enable placement with the correct instrumentation. An implant mount serves to facilitate the delivery of a dental implant to surgical site, and it may be used to rotate implant to correct depth. The implant mount is then removed from the implant to obtain visual confirmation of the position. Other implant systems incorporate a direct-drive feature, in which an instrument engages directly into implant, allowing for a simpler procedure and better vision during implant placement.

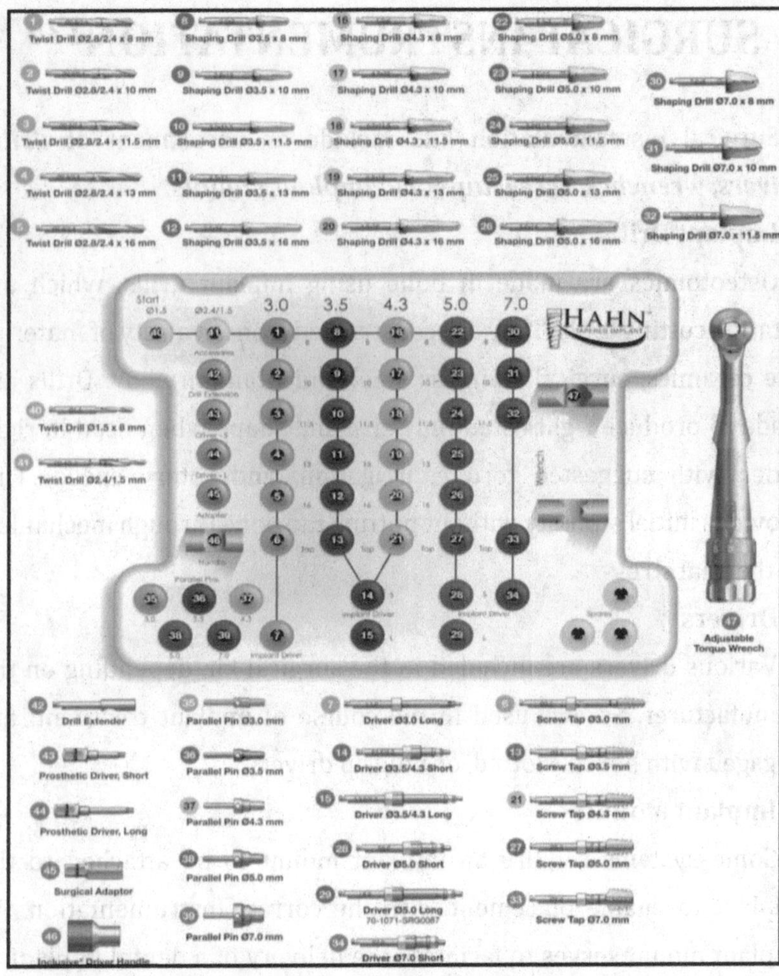

Fig.29 - Hahn implant surgery kit with various components. (Prismatik Dentalcraft, Irvine, California.)

Wrenches

Surgical kits include a ratchet wrench or ***torque wrench*** to place the implant. A torque wrench or torque driver is a manual instrument used to apply a specific amount of torque when placing an implant or prosthetic screw. A ***torque controller*** refers to an electronic machine designed for the same purpose. A torque wrench is recommended to ensure the application of a force that conforms to the manufacturer's recommendation.

Implant Components

The ***cover screw,*** sometimes called a ***healing screw,*** is a component used to occlude the connection of the implant while submerged during a two-stage procedure.

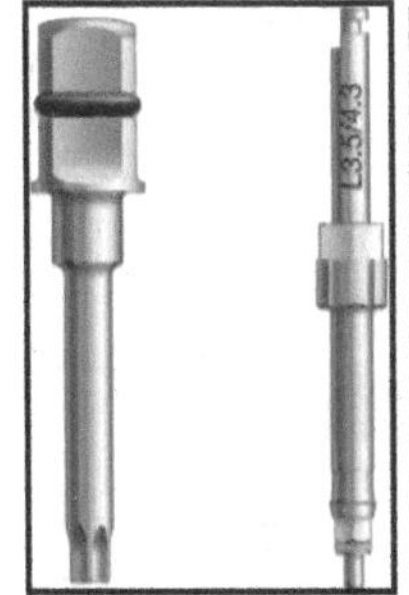

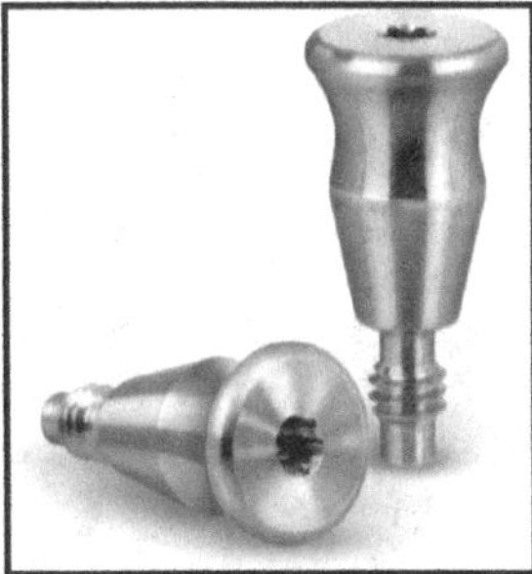

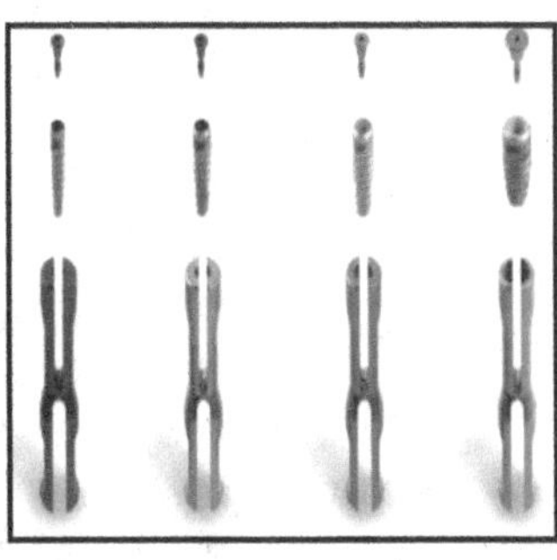

Fig.30 - Hand driver (left) and rotary driver	Fig.31 - Stock/standardized healing abutments	Fig.32 - Hahn implant with holder and cover screw

Guided Surgery

A ***surgical guide,*** or ***surgical template,*** is a device created for a specific case to assist the surgeon in placing the implants in the intended location. Guided surgery involves use of a guide that directs placement of implant.

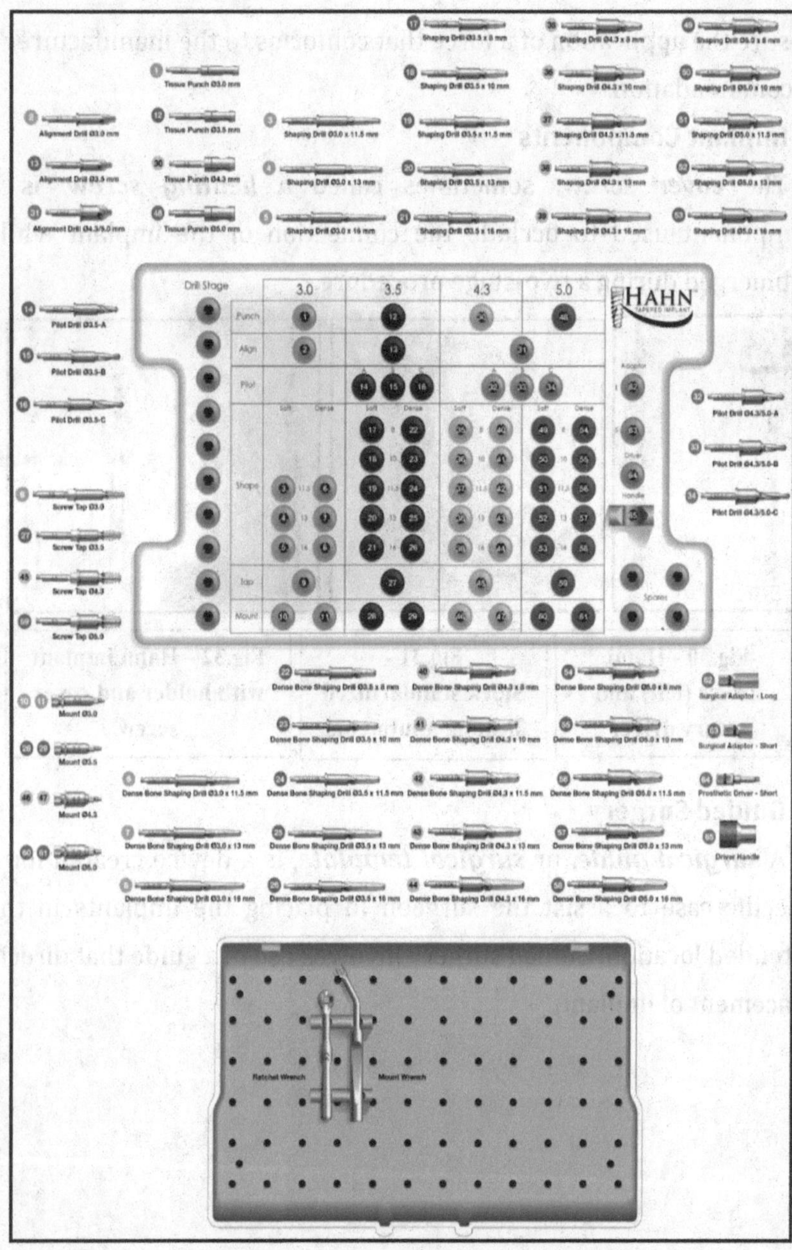

Fig.33 - Hahn guided surgery kit. (Prismatik Dentalcraft, Irvine, California)

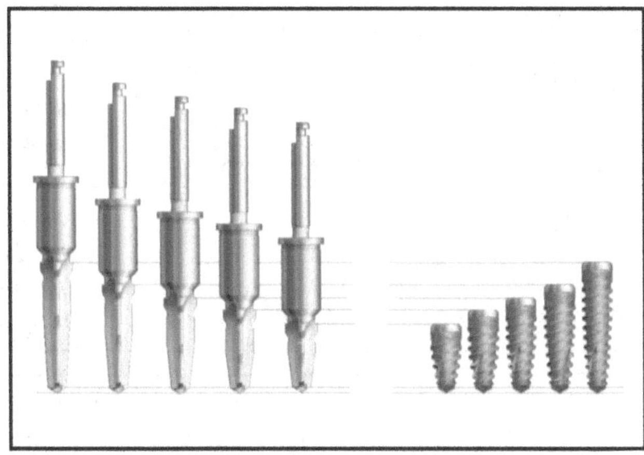

Fig.34 - Hahn-guided surgery drills are designed with a cuff that fits precisely into the guide sleeve and eliminates the need for a spoon to hold the drill in place. Each drill is matched with the corresponding implant height

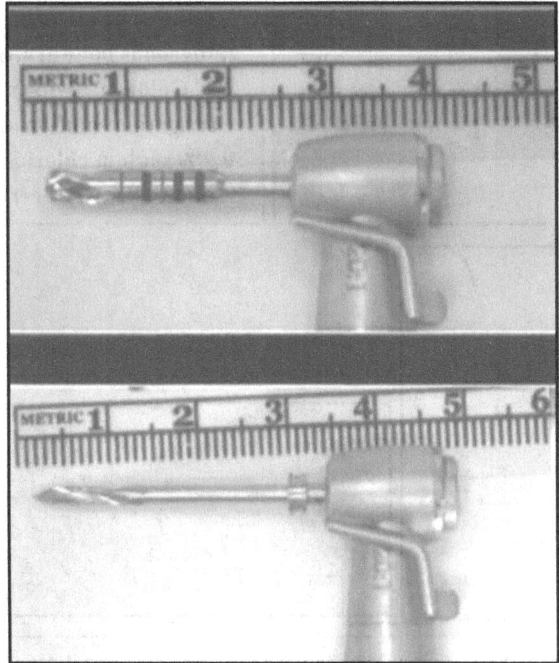

Fig.35 - Standard surgical drill versus guided drill with depth stopper is approximately 10 mm longer

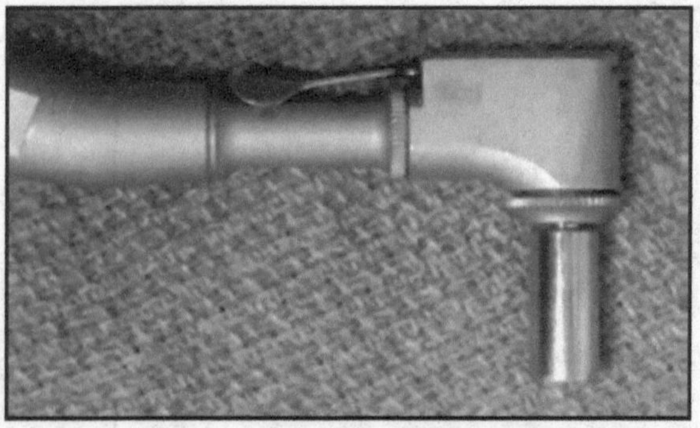

Fig.36 - Slow-speed latch-type handpiece used to remove tissue. Tissue punch bur which corresponds to the diameter of the intended implant size

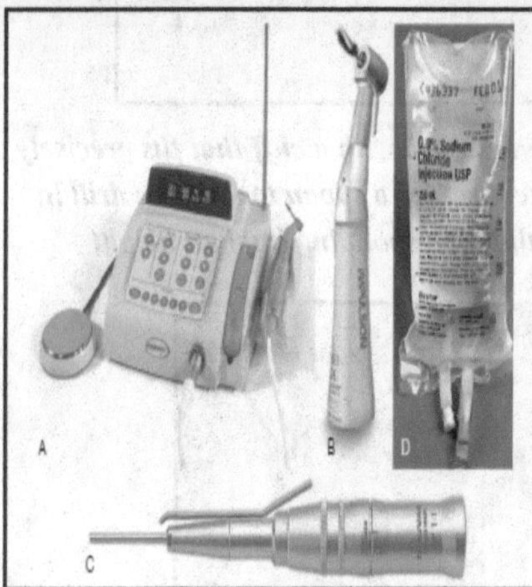

Fig.37 - Aseptico surgical motor (Aseptico, Woodinville, Wash.). 20:1 reduction handpiece for drilling osteotomy and placing implants (Aseptico). 1:1 handpiece that is used for bone removal or harvesting autogenous bone grafts (Nouvag, Goldach, Switzerland). Irrigation solution should be 0.9% sodium chloride or sterile saline. (Baxter, Deerfield, Ill.)

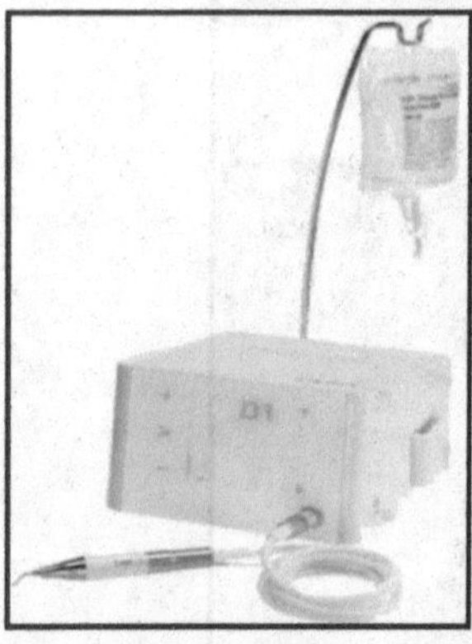

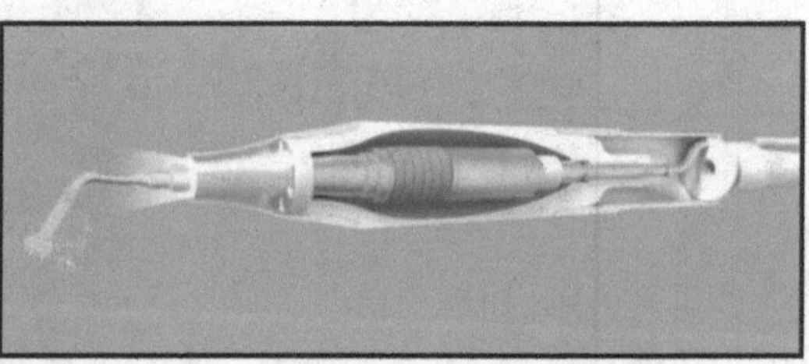

Fig. 38 - Piezo surgery motor console (Salvin, Charlotte, N.C.) Vibrating handpiece that uses ultrasound frequency technology, resulting in precision and safe cutting of hard tissue

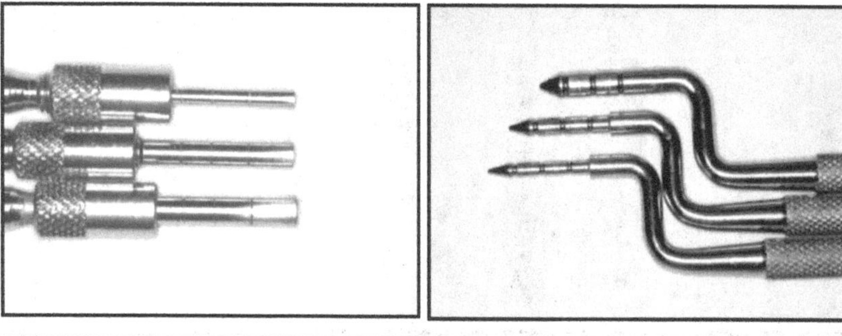

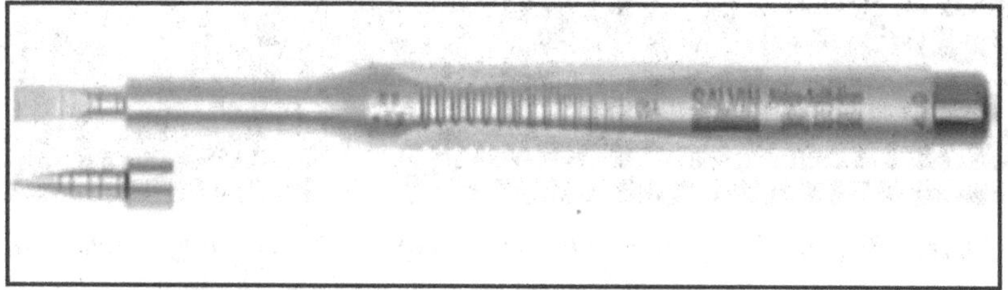

Fig.39 - Osteotomes
Sinus osteotomes with adjustable stops
Offset osteotomes to increase osteotomy diameter
Straight osteotome for bone spreading.

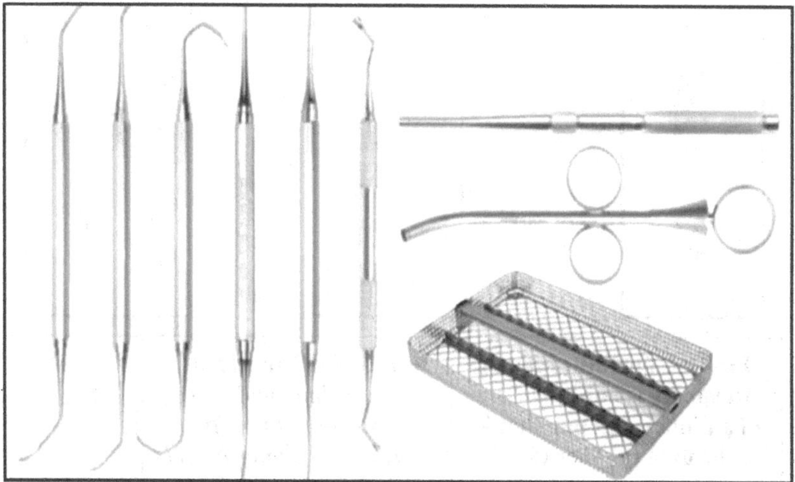

Fig.40 - Basic sinus surgery kit.

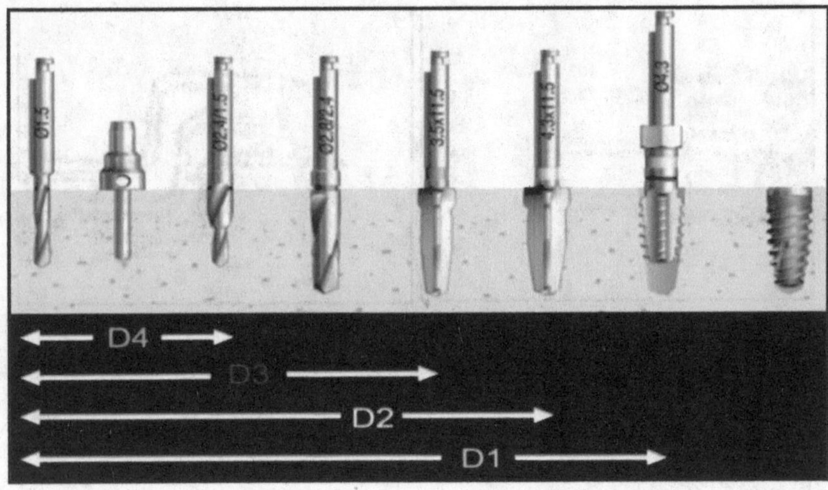

Fig.41 - The number of steps in the preparation of the osteotomy is related to bone density. Usually, D1 will require all drills including the bone tap, the D2 protocol uses all drills except the bone tap, D3 requires the standard protocol stopping at the second to last drill, and D4 uses only the first or second drills.

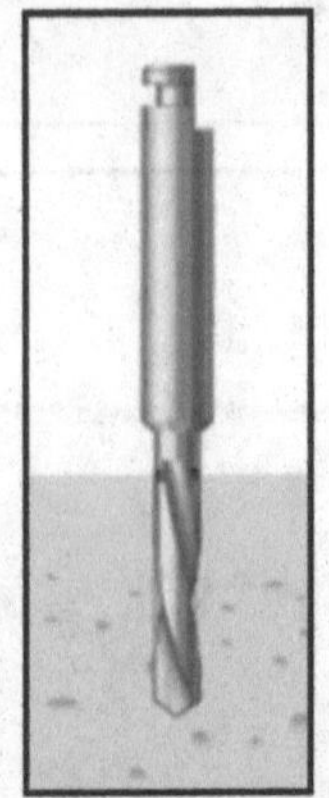

Fig.44 - If modification of osteotomy is indicated, use of a Lindemann bur should be used to reposition osteotomy

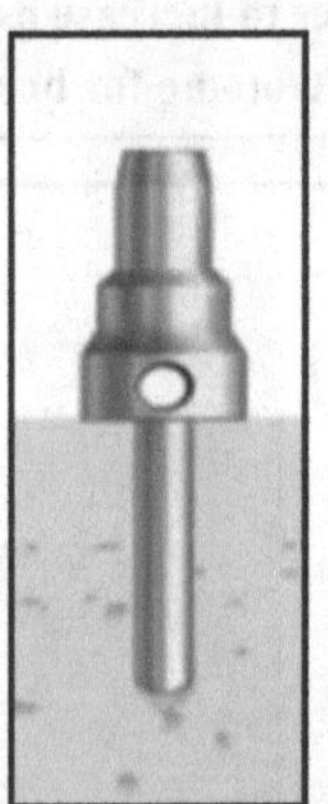

Fig.43 - Parallel pin placed into pilot drill osteotomy to verify positioning clinically and radiographically

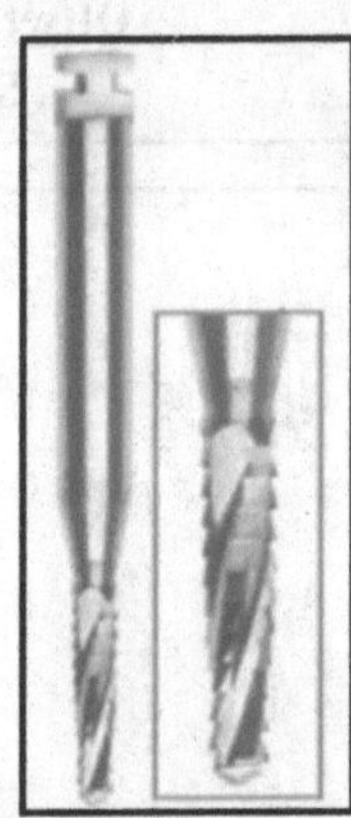

Fig.42 - Pilot drill

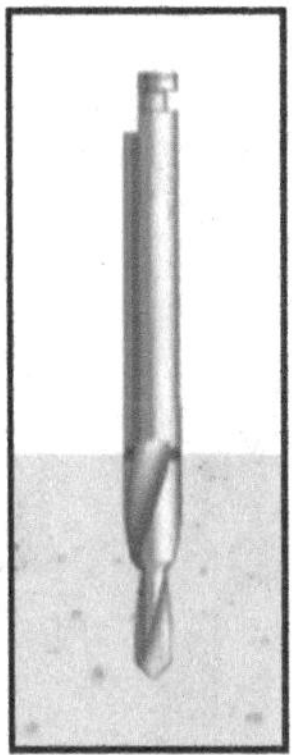

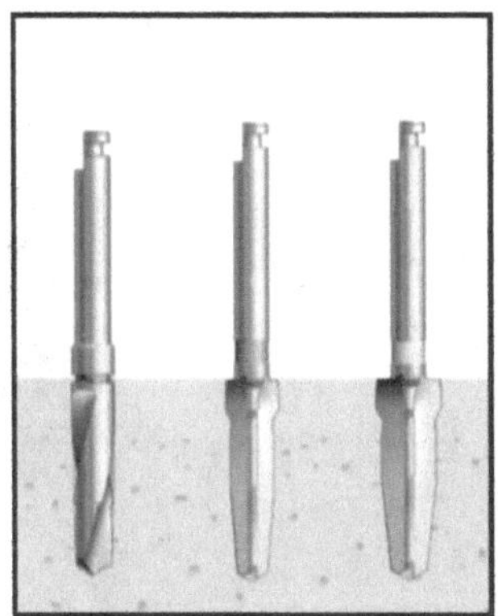

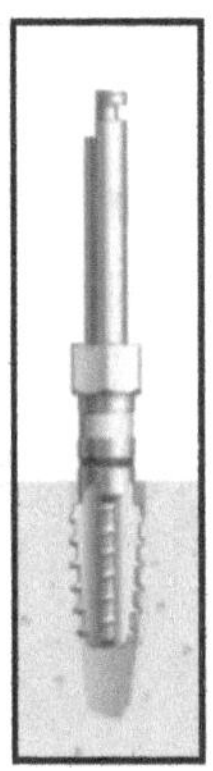

Fig.45 - A second twist drill is used to widen the osteotomy to allow for larger-diameter drills	**Fig.46 - Final drills are used to widen the osteotomy to accommodate the diameter of the intended implant**	***Fig.47 - Tap drill Used mainly in D1 bone at approximately 30 rpm***

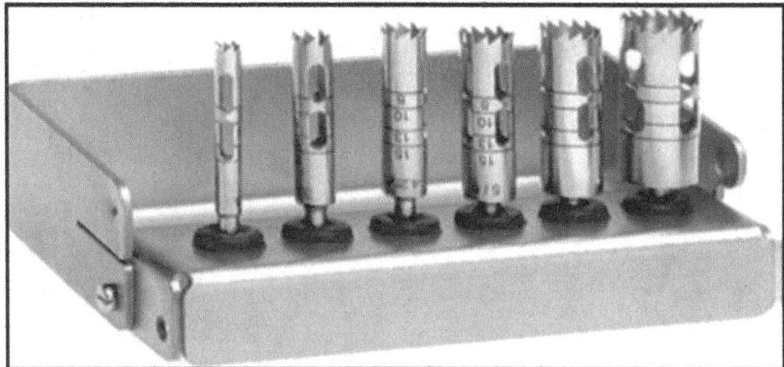

Fig.48 - Trephine burs

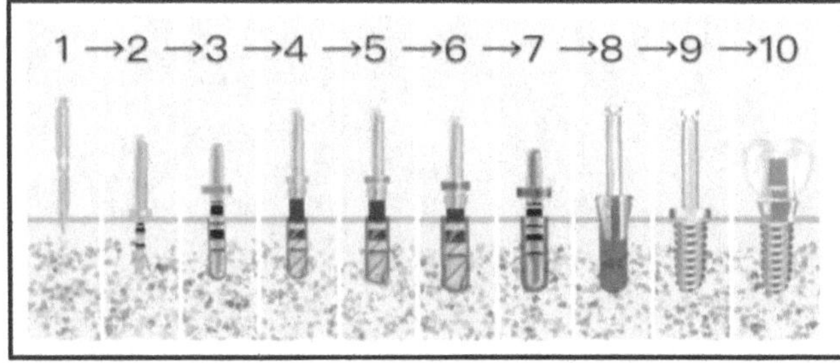

Fig.49 – Conventional multiple drilling sequences

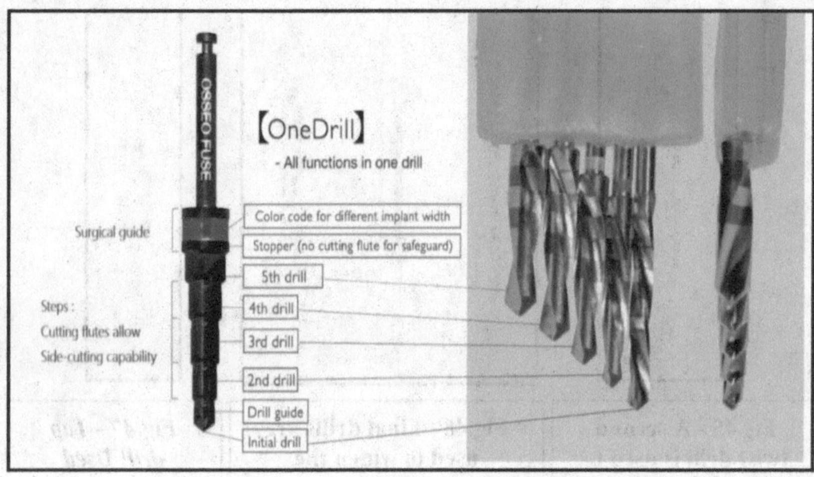

Fig.50 - The OsseoFuse OneDrill® combines the functions of multiple drills into a single drill for use in completing a dental implant osteotomy from start to finish with one drill, including self-tapping.

TECHNIQUES USED IN IMMEDIATE IMPLANT PLACEMENT SURGERY

It is always safe to start with pilot drill due to palatal wall's hardness, since there is a possibility that drill bit will slip into socket & puncture buccal bone plate. Two methods can be employed to steer clear of this issue.[109]

1. Round bur technique: A small round bur that is roughly one-third of apex on palatal wall of socket is used to start drilling process. After that, it is done while maintaining a palatal orientation concerning tooth axis. This method should be used when there is quick implantation and little to no tissue loss.
2. Trephine technique: Permits improved axis implant control as bone heals for further filling. Utilizing a trephine bur, bone graft can be harvested and subsequently placed between implant and buccal bone socket. To maximize main stability of implant, drilling should be done beyond socket during implant site preparation.

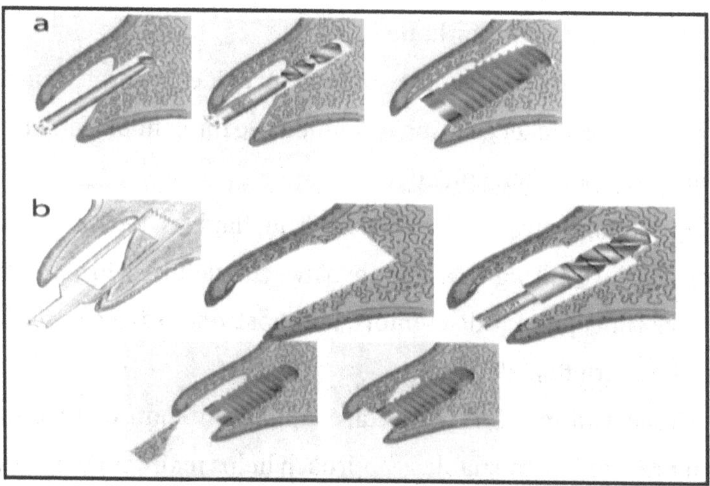

Fig.51 - a: Bur round technique: a1: Trepanation using a bur round; a2: Implant drilling; a3: Implant placement. b: Trepan technique: b1,b2: Bone graft harvesting using a trepan; b3: Implant drilling; b4: Implant placement; b5: Bone graft placement between the implant and buccal bone socket.

IMMEDIATE IMPLANT PLACEMENT USING A FLAPLESS APPROACH

Use of flapless procedure offers an immediate implant placement or socket grafting method for extraction that is less invasive. There is less disruption of arterial supply because interdental papilla is still intact. The implant is inserted using the flapless technique without lifting any flaps. It makes the process easier, cutting down on operating duration and patient discomfort while increasing patient acceptance of implant protocols.[131] Complications like fenestration and bony dehiscence do exist, though. According to a clinical study, flapless surgery has a 4.73% dehiscence rate.[132] From a biological perspective, primary benefit of a flapless technique is maintenance of arterial supply to alveolar bone through preservation periosteum and supraperiostal. According to certain clinical research, flapless surgery may be able to stop minor bone loss.[133]

The flapless technique can indeed provide several benefits in certain cases of socket grafting or immediate implant placement. Here are some key points to consider:[1]

1. Minimally invasive approach: The flapless technique avoids raising flaps, resulting in a less invasive procedure. This can reduce operative time, patient discomfort, and post-operative complications associated with flap elevation.

2. Preservation of interdental papilla: By not disturbing the interdental papilla, the flapless approach helps maintain blood supply

to surrounding tissues. This may contribute to improved healing and preservation of soft tissue esthetics.

3. Simplified procedure: The flapless technique simplifies the surgical procedure by eliminating the need for flap reflection and suturing. This can streamline the process, making it more efficient and potentially more appealing for patients.

4. Preservation of periosteum and blood supply: By preserving the periosteum and supraperiosteal blood supply, the flapless technique can help maintain the vitality of the alveolar bone. This may contribute to better healing outcomes and potentially prevent marginal bone loss.

5. Complications: While the flapless technique offers advantages, it is important to consider potential complications associated by this approach, like bony dehiscence and fenestration. Careful case selection, appropriate patient assessment, and proper surgical technique are essential to minimize these risks.

Extraction, immediate implant placement, and guided bone regeneration using a flapless approach

Barry K. Bartee, DDS, MD

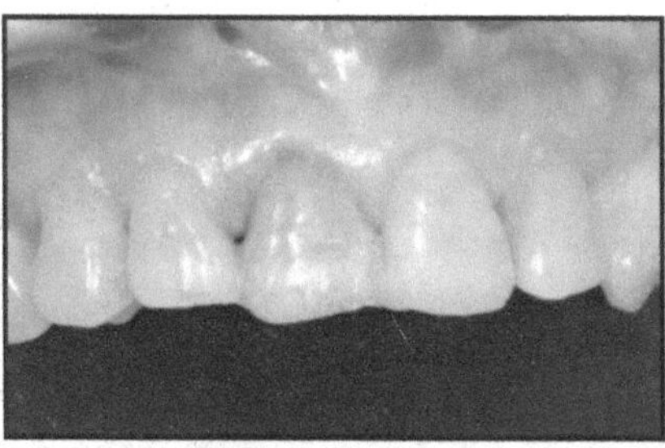

Fig.52 - 60-year-old female presented with a crown-root fracture of a non-vital maxillary right central incisor. The crown was temporarily stabilized with a composite resin bonded to the adjacent teeth

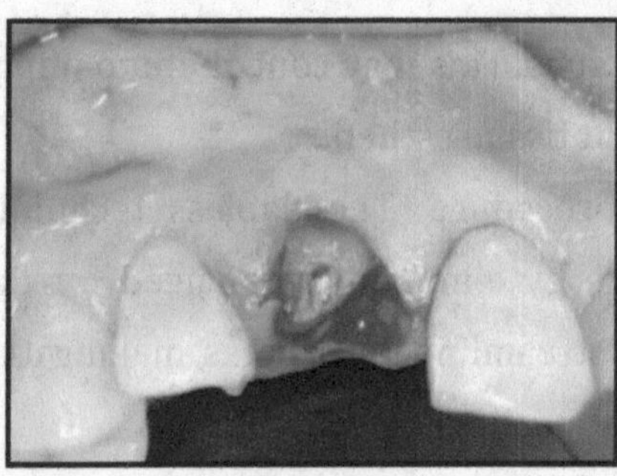

Fig.53 - Extraction of the tooth and immediate implant placement was planned. To minimize soft and hard tissue recession, a flapless, minimally invasive extraction technique was employed

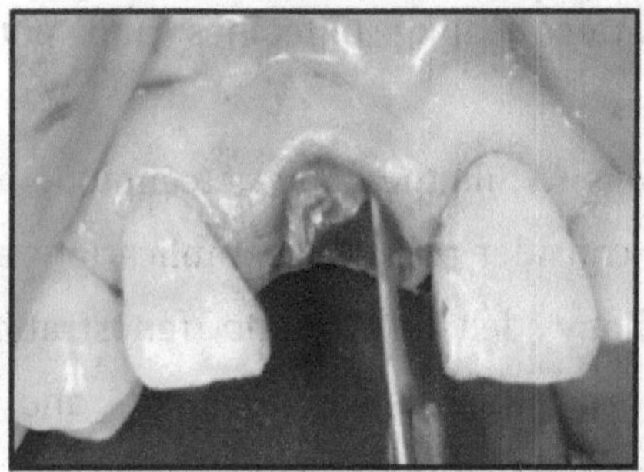

Fig.54 - The tooth root was extracted using only an intrasulcular incision. A #15 blade was used to sever the periodontal ligament and create space for root luxation and elevation

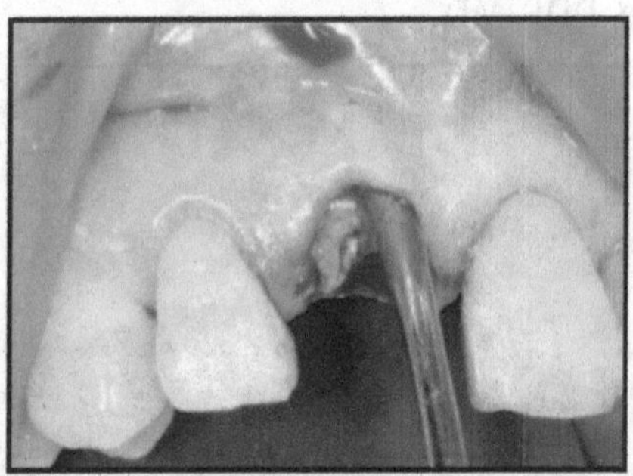

Fig.55 - Next, a subperiosteal pocket was created on the buccal and palatal aspect of the socket using a micro periosteal elevator.

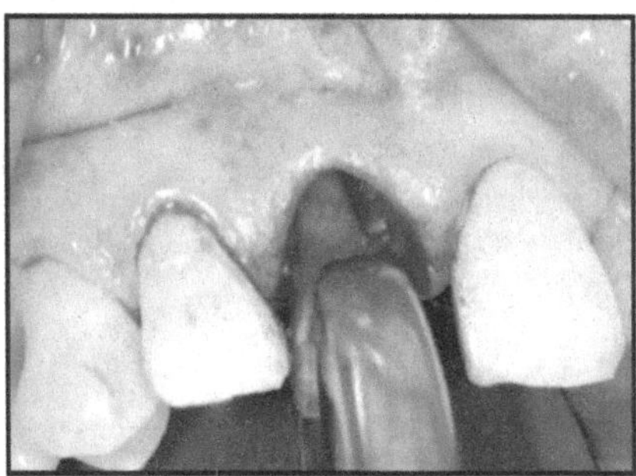

Fig.56 - Following luxation and initial elevation of the root with the micro elevator, the tooth was removed with forceps.

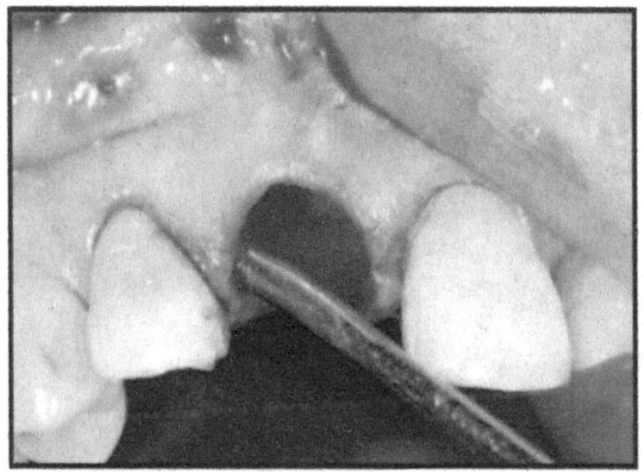

Fig. 57 - The interdental papillae were carefully undermined and elevated. This can be done with a small periosteal elevator or curette.

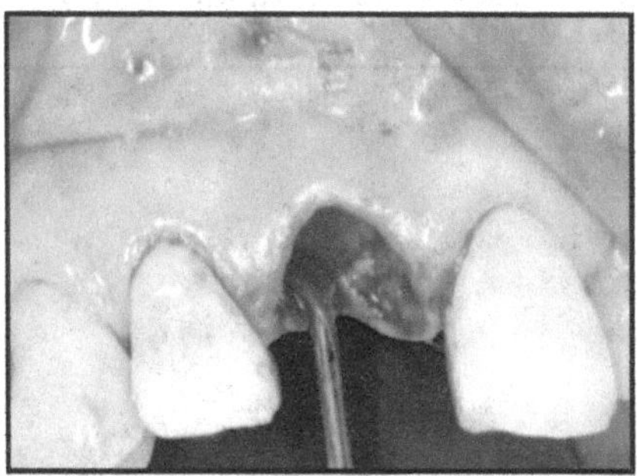

Fig. 58 - All remaining soft tissue was removed from the interior and margins of the socket with a sharp curette

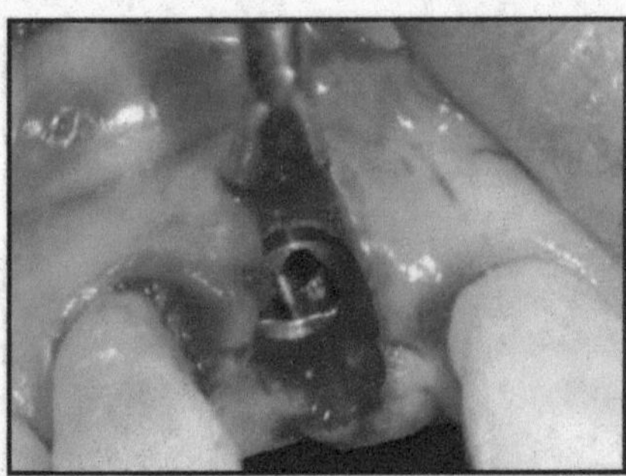

Fig. 59 - The implant osteotomy was done in the standard fashion, with the implant being placed against the palatal wall of the socket.

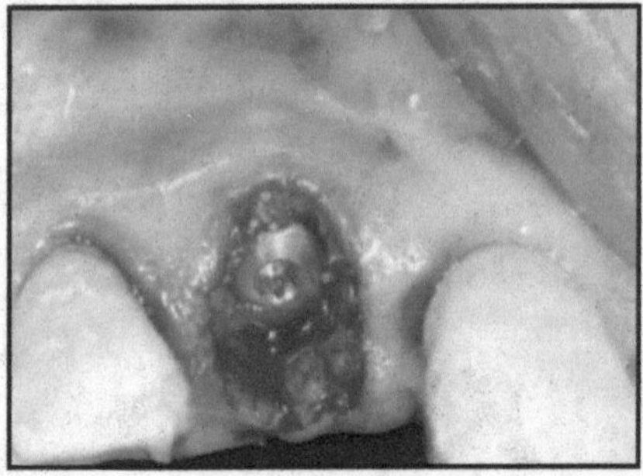

Fig. 60 - The gap between the facial aspect of the implant and the buccal wall was filled with a combination of autogenous bone chips harvested from the implant osteotomy combined with allograft bone

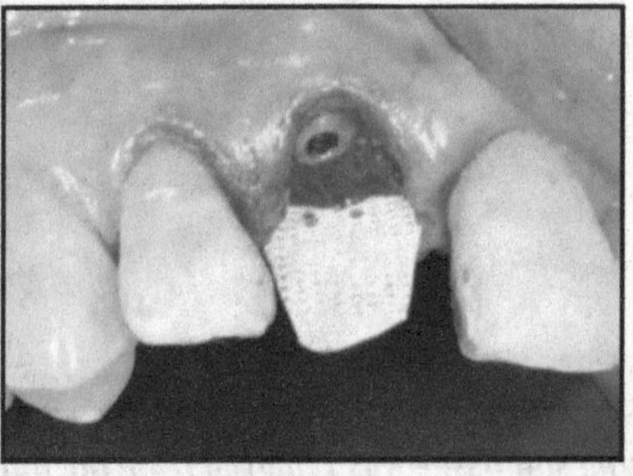

Fig. 61 - A textured, high-density PTFE barrier membrane (Cytoplast® TXT-200) is placed. The membrane is trimmed and then placed into the superiosteal pocket on the palatal aspect

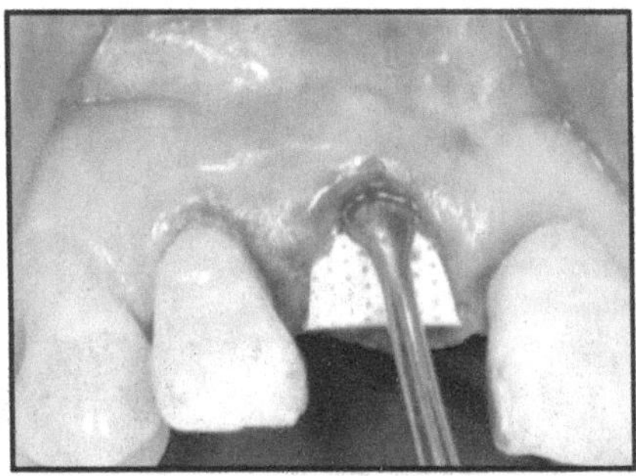

Fig. 62 - The membrane is then tucked under the facial flap.

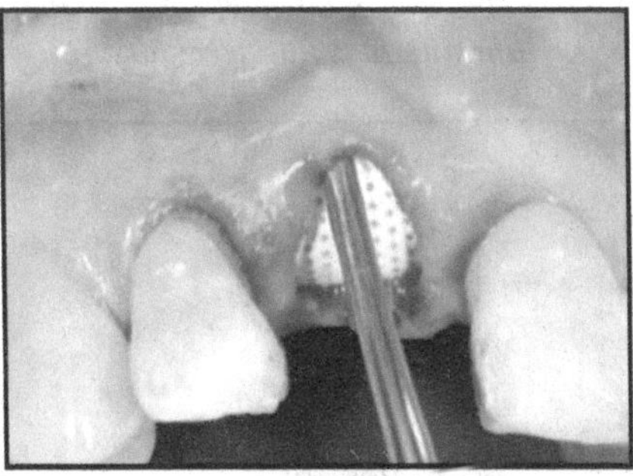

Fig. 63 - Next, the membrane is tucked under the interdental papillae, taking care to keep the edge of the material a minimum of 1.0 mm away from adjacent tooth roots

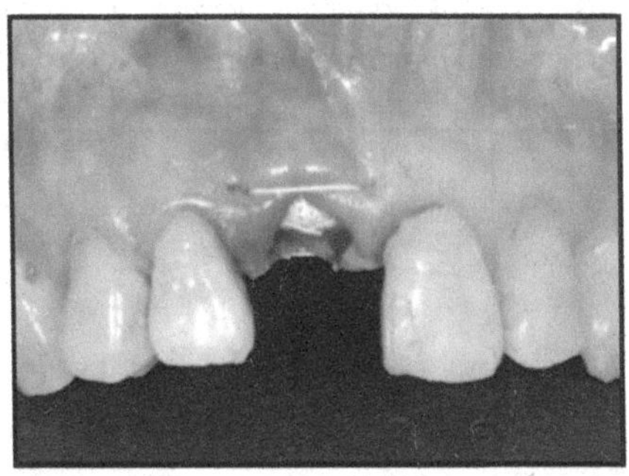

Fig. 64 - A single 3-0 suture (Cytoplast® PTFE Suture; CS0518) is placed to further stabilize the membrane. The membrane is intentionally left exposed, as primary closure is not required in this technique

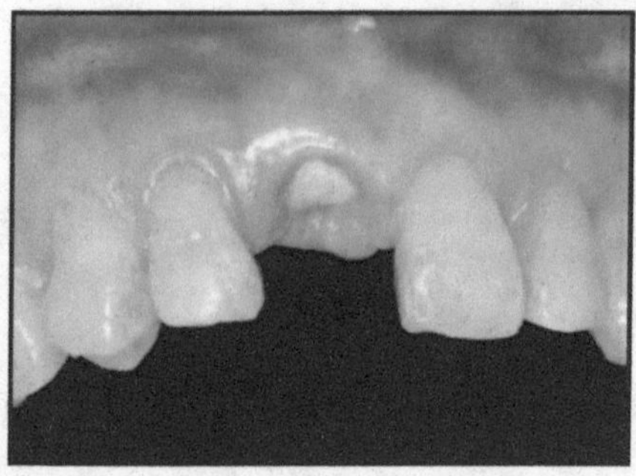

Fig. 65 - The surgical site at 3 weeks. The exposed membrane is easily removed by grasping with a tissue forceps. Topical anesthesia may be used, but local anesthesia is not necessary.

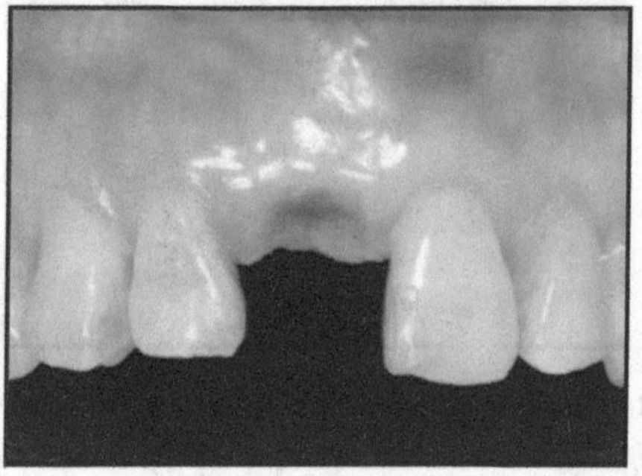

Fig.66 - The site at 6 weeks after implant placement (three weeks after membrane removal), reveals keratinized mucosa forming across the former extraction site.

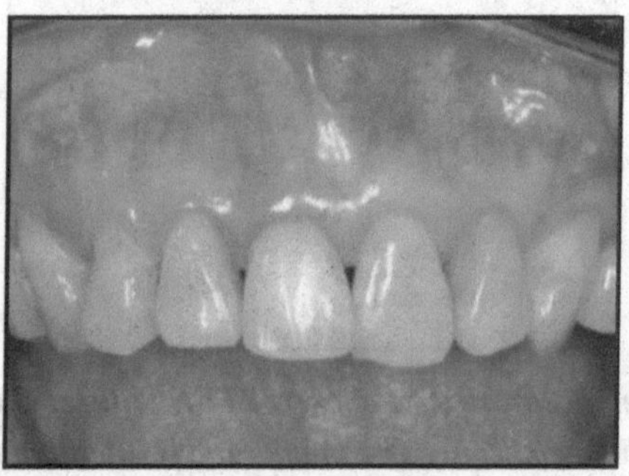

Fig.67 - The clinical view following placement of the implant abutment and acrylic provisional restoration.

THE RULE OF 5 TRIANGLES:[1]

The 5 key aspects to consider when placing immediate implants are:

1. Presence of a buccal plate: Buccal bone plate plays a critical role in maintaining aesthetics of implant site. It is important to assess thickness or integrity of buccal plate before deciding on immediate implant placement.
2. Primary stability: Achieving this is essential for success of immediate implants. Primary stability refers to initial mechanical stability of implant
3. Implant design: Design of implant can impact its stability and integration with the surrounding tissues. Self-tapered implants are often preferred for immediate placement as they can enhance primary stability by compressing alveolar bone during insertion.
4. Filling gap between buccal plate and implant: gap and distance between buccal bone and implant should be restored with biomaterial to promote formation of bone and prevent soft tissue recession. This can help maintain the aesthetics of the implant site and minimize complications.
5. Tissue biotype: Thickness and quality of gingival tissues, known as tissue biotype, can influence aesthetic outcome of immediate implants. Thicker gingival biotype is generally more favorable as it provides better support and stability for the soft tissues around the implant.

INCISION DESIGNS[1]

When placing implant in aesthetic zone, it is essential to employ conservative flap designs for minimizing tissue trauma and preserve aesthetics of surrounding soft tissue. Here are some considerations for flap design:

1. Full-thickness flap design: A full-thickness flap design is used instead of flapless procedure. This allows for better visualization and access to the underlying structures during implant placement. It provides more control over the surgical site and allows for adequate management of the soft tissue.
2. Flapless technique: A flapless technique should only be considered in specific cases where is favorable zone of attached gingiva, low aesthetic demand, radiographic assessment indicates favorable conditions, like thick and intact facial bony walls. However, it is generally recommended to use a flap design to ensure proper visualization and control during the procedure.
3. Vertical releasing incision: For gaining access for site and inspect buccal plate any fenestration & dehiscence defect, vertical releasing incision can be made into the mesial/ distal papilla. This incision allows for better exposure and assessment of buccal bone, which is crucial for implant placement in aesthetic zone.

Bilateral incision designs: In cases flap advancement is desired for submerged or semi-submerged approach of healing, bilateral incision designs can be employed. This is particularly important in aesthetic zone for allowing over-contouring of buccal profile using soft and hard tissue grafting. Use of bilateral incisions facilitates flap advancement and better control over the final aesthetic outcome.

COMPLICATIONS

Immediate implant placement is frequently the preferred treatment for tooth replacement following extraction due to several advantages. These include reduced treatment time, decreased surgical procedures, lower morbidity, and the potential for immediately delivering a provisional prosthesis following the extraction. These benefits collectively lead to increased patient satisfaction. Additionally, survival rates for this approach similar for early & delayed implant placement modalities.[134]

Most common complications which occur with immediate implant placement after extraction of natural tooth include [135]:-

- Poor implant positioning
- Membrane exposure during healing
- Inadequate bands of keratinised tissue after healing
- Gingival recession
- Implant failure
- Unacceptable esthetic outcomes.
- **POOR IMPLANT POSITIONING** [136]

Malpositioned implants may lead to significant complications in loss of peri-implant recession and soft tissue volume of its papillae or mucosa, might complicate successful prosthodontic rehabilitation. At Third ITI Consensus Conference 2003 in Gstaad, Switzerland, concept of "danger" & "comfort" zones to position implants in aesthetic site was established.[137]

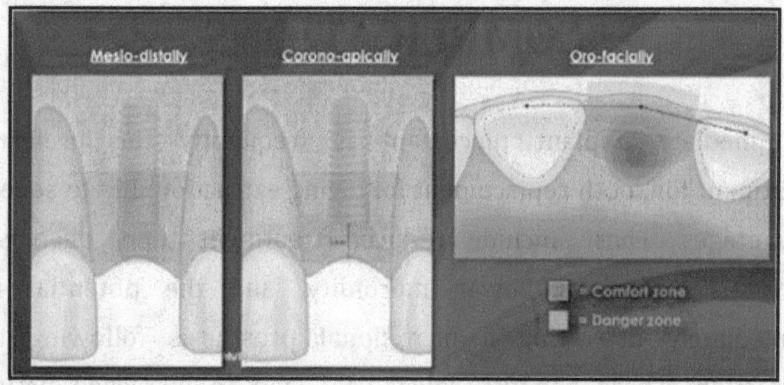

Fig. 68 - Comfort and danger zones for positioning of implants in three dimensions: mesiodistally, Corono-apically, and Orofacially.

- **Mesiodistal malposition**

Placing an implant close to a neighbouring tooth can result in reduced tissue height between the tooth and the implant, potentially leading to bone resorption in the neighbouring area. Additionally, a micro space at implant-abutment junction can induce localized bone remodelling, causing saucer-like defect in bone surrounding the implant. This defect may manifest in a circular pattern and could result in bone loss if bone wall is thin. Proper positioning of implant, more than 1.5 mm away to neighbouring tooth, can mitigate these issues. However, positioning the implant less than 1.5 mm from adjacent tooth may lead to bone loss, affecting tissue height and potentially causing gum recession and exposure of neighbouring tooth's root surface.

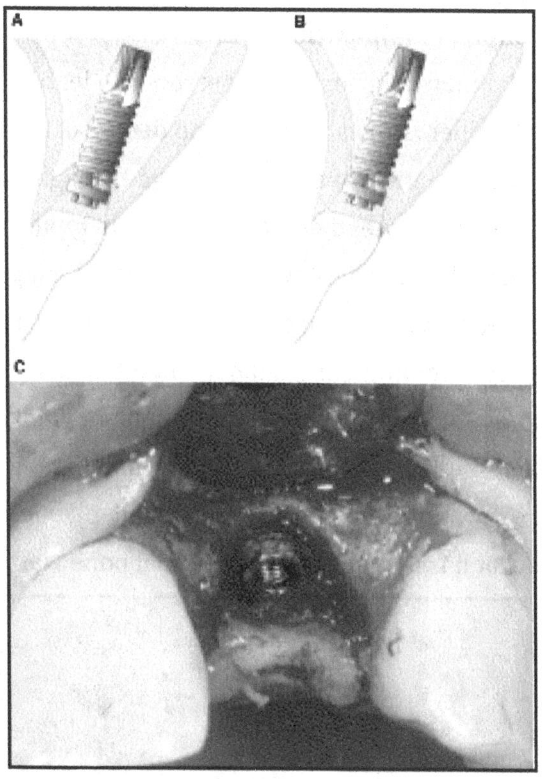

Fig. 69 - The formation of a crater- or saucer-like defect around implants with an external hexagon connection.

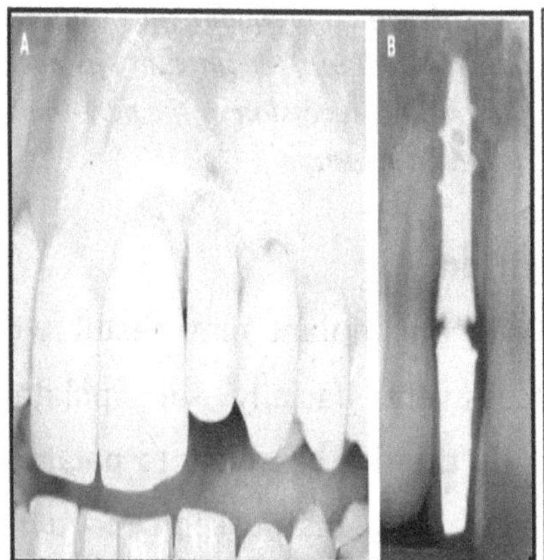

Fig. 70 -The papilla between the maxillary left central incisor and the lateral incisor implant has reduced in height. In addition, there has been recession of the gingiva on the distal and disto-facial aspect of the central incisor. the radiograph shows the proximity of the implant to the maxillary left central incisor. The peak of bone on the distal aspect of the tooth has receded

- **Coronoapical malposition**

The vertical dimension, positioning errors can lead to discomfort if the implant shoulder is too shallow or too deep. To achieve a natural appearance, the implant crown must emerge through soft tissue cuff in appropriate contour. Aesthetic zone, implants typically positioned somewhat palatally to align with restoration's cingulum, which requires sufficient vertical and horizontal distance. A required vertical distance from implant shoulder to midfacial mucosal margin is 3-4 mm to avoid visibility of the abutment or implant shoulder. Deeply placed implants, common with immediate implants, can complicate restoration and impact control of plaque, especially if extraction socket has damaged and thin facial bone wall.

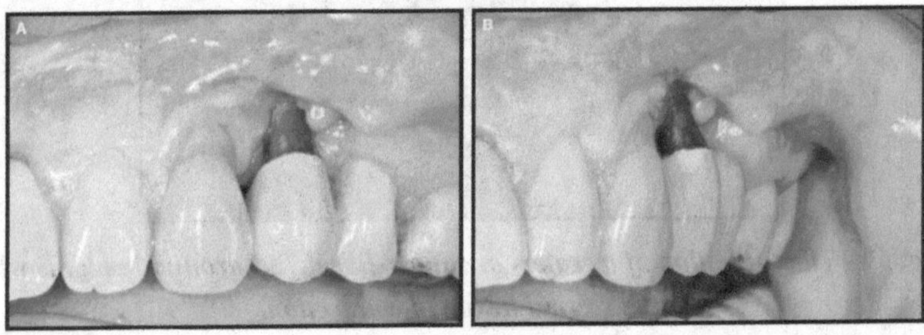

Fig. 71 - A and B, The implant in the maxillary first premolar site has been placed with the shoulder too far coronally. In addition, the implant has been placed with a slight facial malposition. The result is recession of the peri-implant mucosa and an aesthetic disaster

- **Orofacial and axial malposition**

Defects of orofacial positioning in an implant may result while implant being positioned excessively facially or palatally. Additionally, implants may be axially tilted excessively to palatal or facial side. Axial malposition and orofacial malposition frequently coexist. An implant positioned too far palatally due to pre-existing bone loss might occur. This is an unusual consequence. When facial aspect's tissue volume is deficient, palatal implant misplacement might result in markedly unfavorable cosmetic consequences.

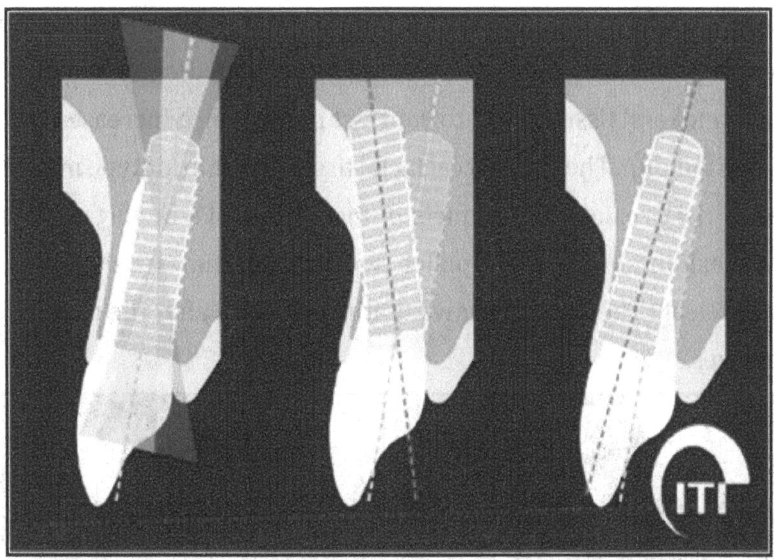

Fig. 72 - Diagrammatic representation of facial and axial malposition of implants that result in the implant shoulder being positioned in the facial and palatal danger zones, respectively. [138]

❖ MEMBRANE EXPOSURE DURING HEALING [135]

Membrane exposure during process of healing was common, with its significance dependent on the type of membrane used, essential for ensuring primary flap closure for most membrane systems. It is advised to advance flaps correctly, without strain, and to use suture material to hold them at place during early phases of healing. Results is usually unaffected by exposure to absorbable membranes such as collagen membranes or Polyglactin 910 (Vicryl, Ethicon; Johnson and Johnson, Somerville, NJ, USA). Bacterial growth over polyglactin 910 membrane is negligible and it breaks down in an acidic state.

Flap advancement is not necessary for these membranes to cover since essential in their success. When flaps are not advanced, there is often adequate keratinized tissue remaining between initial flap edges after membrane dissolves. But, in some situations—like those involving smokers—still wise to advance flap despite membrane since smokers' tissues tend to contract more, which increases risk of plaque buildup. The thin buccal facial tissue of a thin biotype may melt due to the breakdown products of membrane. It's important to use chlorhexidine on a cotton pellet two or three times a day to keep region clean. There will be new keratinized tissue after the membrane dissolves.

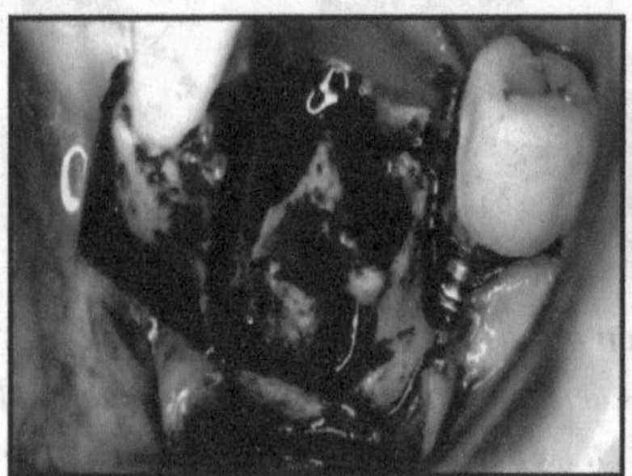

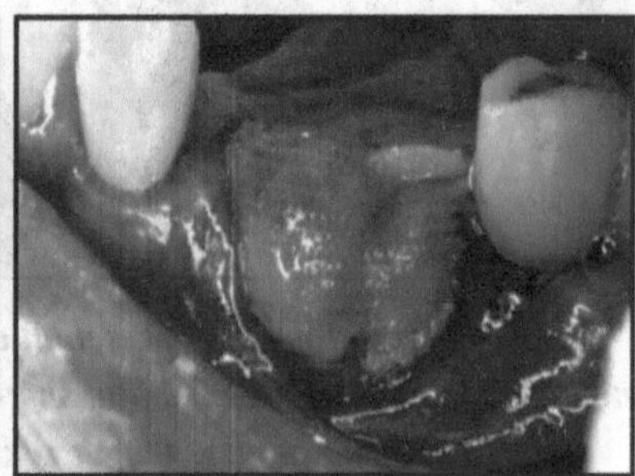

Fig. 73 - Significant bone loss is seen. The area is grafted with cortical freeze-dried bone and covered with a Vicryl membrane. The membrane breakdown product dissolves the thin buccal soft tissue.

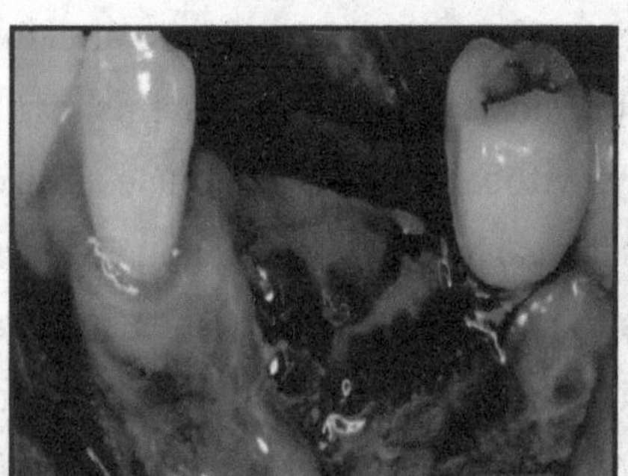

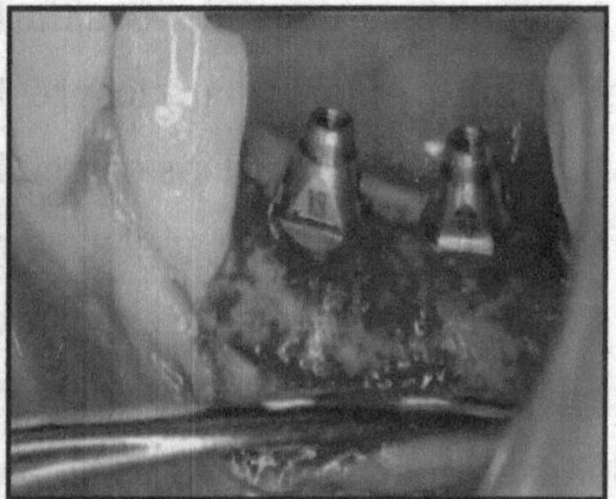

Fig. 74 - As the membrane dissolves islands of keratinized tissue can be seen. At implant placement, new bone growth can be observed.

❖ INADEQUATE BANDS OF KERATINISED TISSUE AFTER HEALING

Zigdon & Machtei (2008)[139], **Schrott, Jimenez et.al (2009)**[140], **Boynueğri, Nemli & Kasko (2013)**[141] Studied importance of keratinised tissue around implants. They mentioned that keratinised mucosa around implants acts like barrier against subgingival plaque & microorganism thatcould harm dental implants' biological success.

A minimum 2mm width of keratinised mucosa, in that 1 mm be attached for achieving proper gingival health was recommended by **Lang and Löe** in **1972.**[142]

Kungsadalpipob et al. (2020) examined relationship between lack of keratinized mucosa & health of peri-implant tissue. Findings observed a strong correlation between higher mucosal recession, plaque deposition, interproximal bone level > 3 mm, & peri-implantitis with absence of keratinized mucosa. These results provide credence to theory that non-keratinized mucosa may be more susceptible to injury in implant-mucosa interface, which might facilitate development. Plaque buildup is three times higher in implants without keratinized mucosa than that have it.[143] When keratinized mucosa is absent, environment may be harder to maintain and more prone to mechanical irritation and discomfort during normal dental cleanings.[144]

❖ GINGIVAL RECESSION

The risk of gingival recession surrounding implants positioned using an IIP protocol is often increased when implants are positioned too close to the labial surface or when broad implants are used, approaching the labial bone with minimal "gap" area. Sustaining an implant requires enough labial space for long-term upkeep.[135]

In locations where dental implants were placed right away, apical migration of free mucosal margin surrounding implants was frequent. It has been connected to a number of things, including:

✓ **Three-dimensional (3-D) bone-to-implant relationship regarding the mesiodistal, buccolingual and apical-coronal position.**[145] - Maintaining distance of 1-4 mm from external bone surface implant shoulder is recommended for stable aesthetic outcomes. Adding bone grafts in sites of more than 1 mm of horizontal gap between implant & socket walls minimizes soft tissue alterations around immediate implants. Chances of mid-facial mucosal recession is 3 times higher around immediate implants placed in buccal shoulder position compared with those placed more palatally.

✓ **Tissue biotype & width of keratinised mucosa.** - Patients with thin biotypes were believed to have narrow or long teeth & greater susceptibilities to gingival recession comparing to thick biotypes.[146] Lack of Keratinised Mucosa was critical factor impacting plaque accumulation, mucosal recession, and peri-implant inflammation.[147]

✓ **Thickness of facial bone wall** - Predicting buccal plate's resorption requires knowledge about thickness of bone. Therefore, for initial implant implantation, buccal plate thickness with at least 2 mm is preferable to compensate for bone loss during healing.[148]

❖ IMPLANT FAILURE

Implant survival rate is similar to Immediate and delayed placement protocol.[149] There are 2 types of dental implant failure: early and late. An implant exhibiting mobility before final prosthesis is referred to as early implant failure. Within 1-3 years, late implant failure happens.[150]

Causes of early failure	Causes of late failure
Poor bone quantity & quality, systemic diseases such as AIDS, uncontrolled diabetes mellitus, osteoporosis, medications like infection, corticosteroids and bisphosphonates,lack of primary stability, smoking, surgical trauma	Excessive loading, peri-implantitis, bruxism, retained subgingival dental cement, grinding of teeth during night,inadequate prosthetic construction, traumatic occlusion

Dental implant failure is classified based upon local and systemic factors as well.[151]

- Local factors - common or preventable reason of implant failure is infection. In some point during implant therapy, a bacterial infection can occur and lead to implant failure. Word "peri-implantitis" denotes to inflammatory reaction accompanied by loss of bone in soft tissues around implants. It also appears that majority of soft tissue issues, including mucosal abscesses, fistulas, and hyperplastic mucositis, have an infectious cause.
- Systemic factors - The risk factors for implant failure include age, smoking, bruxism, diabetes, cardiovascular disorders, and certain medications. Age, smoking, bruxism, and diabetes can affect the osseointegration process. Cardiovascular disorders impact blood flow and oxygen delivery to tissues, hindering the healing process. Systemic corticosteroid therapy can lead to decreased bone density and immunological suppression, affecting the implant's

osseointegration.

❖ UNACCEPTABLE ESTHETIC OUTCOMES [135]

Even when a practitioner follows right Immediate Implant placement methodology, restoration's aesthetic outcome could still be unsatisfactory. As a result, understanding patient's expectations before to insertion is crucial. Prior to implant implantation, patients with high aesthetic standards should consider a tiered or staged method to ridge preservation.

Level of bone between central and lateral incisors in case provided below appears to be reduced. Although implant seemed to be well positioned in post-restoration radiograph, clinical results show poor aesthetic outcome. The patient didn't have any functional issues and accepted the aesthetic outcome, but from ideal aesthetic standpoint, the restoration was not successful. Esthetic problem in this case was partly because of bone loss between incisors. Multiple procedures are required for creating proper architecture for final restoration before implant placement.

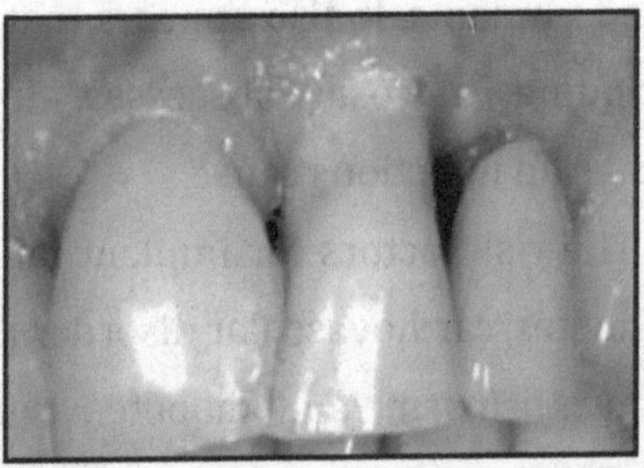

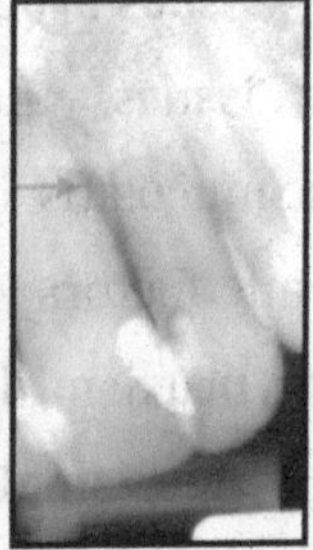

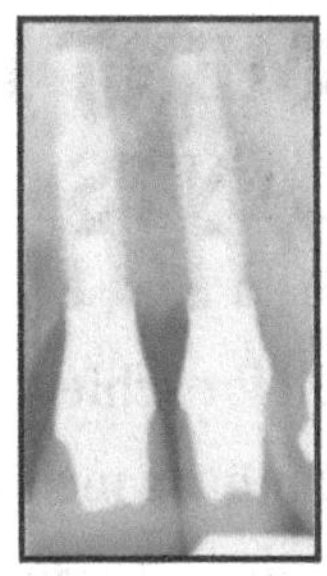

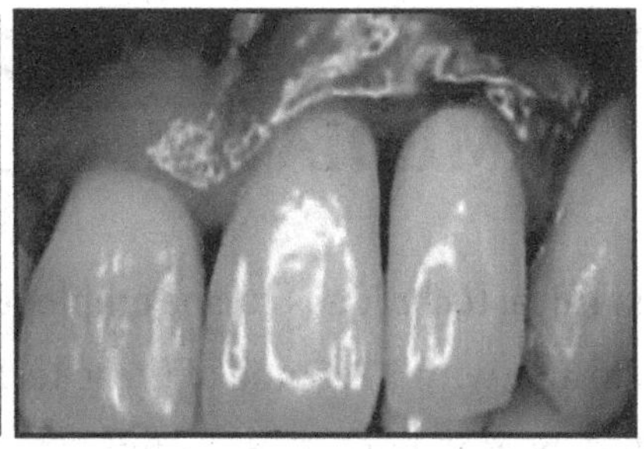

Fig. 75 - (a) Clinical photograph demonstrates the advanced periodontal disease between the central and lateral incisors. (b) Radiograph demonstrating the extent of the bone loss. (c) Radiograph taken of the implant restoration. The implants appear to be in good alignment. (d) Following restoration, a clinical photograph demonstrates the uneven gingival levels on the left central and lateral implants compared to the adjacent teeth.

SOFT TISSUE MANAGEMENT FOR IMMEDIATE IMPLANTS

Various surgical techniques can be employed for achieving primary soft tissue closure with IIP. Some of these techniques include:[1]

1. Rotated buccal flap: This technique involves adjacent tooth rotated buccal flap for achieving closure of soft tissue over implants placed during extraction. It may be used for multiple or single implant sites and can be combined to membrane barriers or grafting materials. However, it requires adequate width of vestibule depth and keratinized mucosa.

2. Connective tissue graft: It can be used for covering immediately placed implants. This technique involves harvesting tissue from the palate or another donor site and grafting it over the implant site. However, the limitation of donor tissue size is a potential challenge with this technique.

3. Acellular dermal matrix allograft: It can be used in combination or alone with grafting materials for covering immediately placed implants. This technique provides an alternative to using autogenous tissue grafts.

4. Gingival grafts: Gingival grafts can also be used to cover immediately placed implants. They can be used alone or in combination with other grafting materials to achieve soft tissue closure.

5. Pediculated flap or Palatal advanced flap: This technique is important in maxillary immediate implant cases. It involves mobilizing tissue from palate and advancing to cover extraction area and implants. This procedure provides good mobility of tissue and

bulk, allowing for accurate coverage of multiple implants and large defect areas. However, secondary healing of the palatal tissue can be prolonged and uncomfortable.

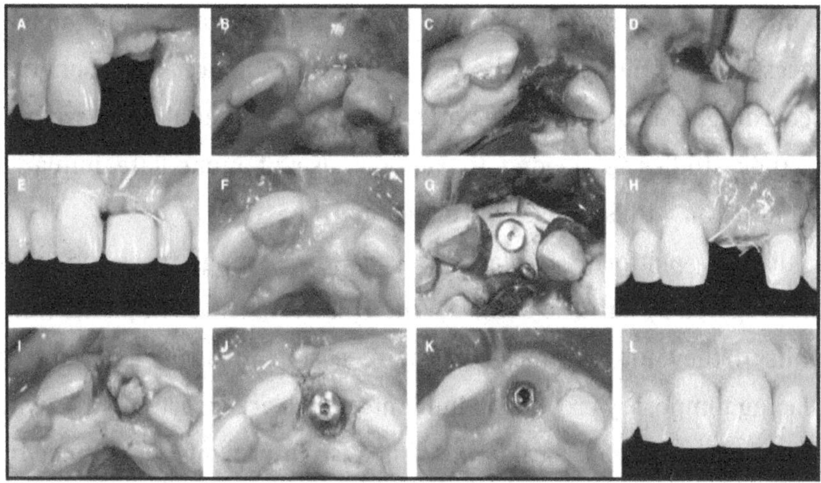

Fig.76

Fig. 76 shows a clinical case of soft tissue management before implant & guided bone regeneration surgery. A-B, Patient's initial situation. C, Minimally-invasive flap combined with tunnelling technique. D, Palatal sub-epithelial connective tissue graft. E, suturing to resin bonded provisional. F, Post-operative healing after 8 weeks. G, Guided bone regeneration simultaneous for implant placement. H, Flap closure with sutures. I, Abutment connection to minimal U-Flap. J, Abutment connection with healing abutment. K, Emergence profile of implant. L, Seven-year follow-up.[152]

Dimensional changes in soft tissue

A soft tissue defect (in width) is observed independently of periodontal biotype, and immediate implant implantation may result in minor gingival recession[153]. In gingiva with thin biotypes and on implants placed buccally, marginal tissue recession is more noticeable.[154] The marginal tissue disparity following immediate implant placement and connective tissue grafts has been smaller than 1 mm.[155] However, using connective tissue grafts to lessen gingival recession has not been shown to have any appreciable benefits, according to a current systematic analysis by Lee et al.[156] Therefore, further studies is needed to support use of immediate implants conjunction with soft tissue transplants.

Use of platform implant switch for setting recession was investigated by **Canullo et al.** [157] When platform switch implants were utilized, they noticed much reduced recession. It has been noted that placing temporary crowns on implants which are inserted right away may help preserve buccal bone while also improving appearance by reducing gingival recession.[158]

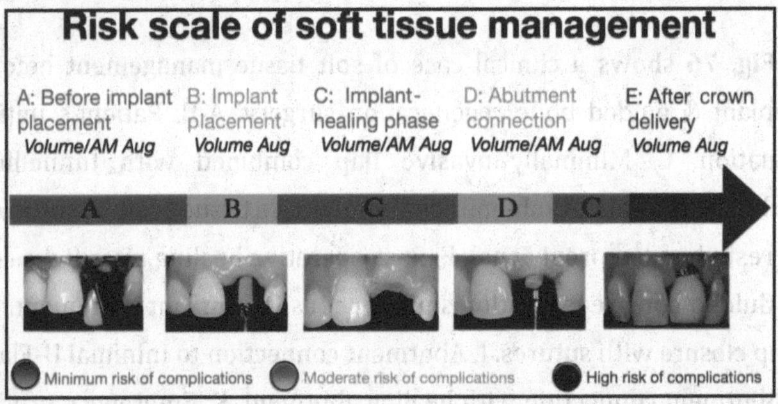

Fig. 77 - Risk scale of soft tissue management before, during, and after implant placement [152] AM, attached mucosa; Aug, augmentation

PLACEMENT OF IMMEDIATE IMPLANT IN INFECTED SITES

In dentistry, dental implants advanced to forefront and were soon norm for oral rehabilitation (Brånemark et al., 1969). Even though conventional have shown long-term success rate with approximately 88% after observation time of 12.2- 23.5 years, protocol of delaying replacement of missing teeth, aesthetics & associated function leads to severe compromise of soft & hard tissue architecture due to rapid bone resorption after tooth loss (**Wilson and Weber, 1993; Hammerle et al., 2004; Chen et al., 2004; Chen and Buser, 2008; Becker et al., 2016**). There are four different implant placement protocols: immediate placement, which entails placing implant in extraction socket right away; early placement, which occurs four to eight weeks after the tooth is extracted; delayed placement, which occurs twelve to sixteen weeks after the tooth is extracted; and late placement, which occurs more than six months after the tooth is extracted. (**Wilson and Weber, 1993; Hammerle et al., 2004**).[159]

Teeth that need to be extracted are typically compromised and frequently infected. The process of bone remodelling may be impacted by infectious process occurring within bony walls of sockets. In these circumstances, fibrous tissue fills in the infected sockets, which ultimately interferes with normal osseous regeneration and wound healing.[160] Numerous suggestions have been made about prompt implantation of implants into diseased sockets, acknowledging that presence of periapical/periodontal infections and disease history are prognostic indicators of implant failure.[161]

In several case studies, **Alsaadi et al.** observed that locations with apical lesions had higher chances of implant failure, particularly in machined surface implants.[162] First case series investigation was carried out by **Pecora et al. (1996)** on 32 titanium implants that were inserted right away into extraction sockets that were contaminated. According to the results, one implant that was inserted into a socket that had an endodontic-periodontic infection failed.[163]

According to research by **Anitua et al. (2016)**, no implant failure was discovered following a 6-year follow-up, suggesting infected sockets are not causative factor for IIP.[164]

Zuffetti et al. (2017), found that three implants which were implanted right away into periodontally/endodontically diseased sites failed, whereas seven implants in non-infected group failed within a year following implant placement.[165] Some researchers have used guided bone regeneration (GBR) and guided tissue regeneration (GTR) procedures with or without plasma rich in growth factors (PRGF) to replace lost bone in infected extraction sockets. These procedures have high success rate, patient satisfaction, and partial preservation of both soft and hard tissues.[160,163,165] Analysis of secondary outcomes (width of keratinized mucosa, clinical attached and bone marginal level surrounding implants) revealed no statistically significant difference between two groups.

Secondary outcome measure's results demonstrate how implants encourage good hard and soft tissue integration.[159]

Curettage of alveolus was done following tooth extraction, prior to implant implantation. A split-mouth dog model, Novaes et al. investigated immediate implantation in ligature-induced periodontitis sites in comparison to healthy controls. Although neither group experienced any failures, control group's BIC was non-significantly higher.[166]

Nine retrospective and prospective studies were combined (control were not included) to determine survival rate of implant inserted in extraction sockets that were infected (**Pecora et al., 1996; Del Fabbro et al., 2003; Casap et al., 2007; Fugazzotto, 2012a; Jofre et al., 2012; Marconcini et al., 2013; Anitua et al., 2016; Velasco-Ortega et al., 2018; Medikeri et al., 2018**). Implants inserted into infected extraction sockets had a 98% survival rate, according to pooled estimate proportion of survival rate, which was 0.98. These results underlined even more how well implants inserted into infected sockets work. According to the meta-analysis's findings, implants placed directly into infected sockets did not differ from implants placed into healthy sites terms of radiological, clinical, or aesthetic aspects surrounding the implants.[159]

According to **Lindeboom et al.**, implants placed immediately had a 92% survival rate while implants placed later had a 100% survival rate. In addition, the group receiving immediately placed implants showed greater buccal marginal tissue recession. The authors hypothesized that an increase keratinized tissue during socket wound healing would explain this.[167] Cultured flora from affected areas indicated Gram-negative organisms that are generally connected to root canal infections. Each study that was reviewed in this review used systemic antibiotics and comprehensive debridement of the socket as part of their treatment protocol. Aggressive antibiotics were utilized in the majority of studies involving newly implanted implants. Antibiotics are thought to be used primarily to reduce bacterial counts before surgery or to minimize any residual infection which was not completely eradicated in time of debridement.

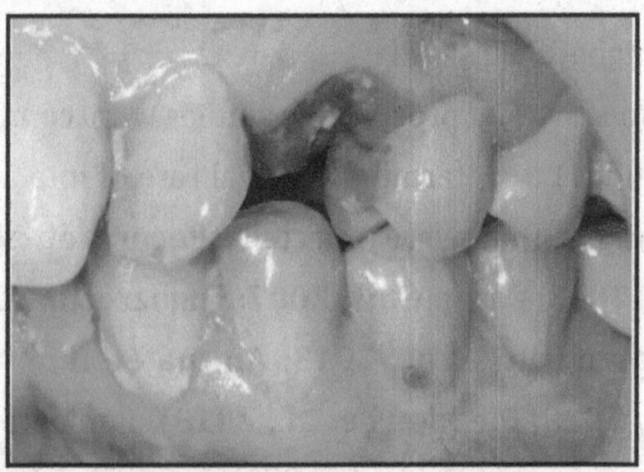

Fig.78 - Preoperative Intraoral View

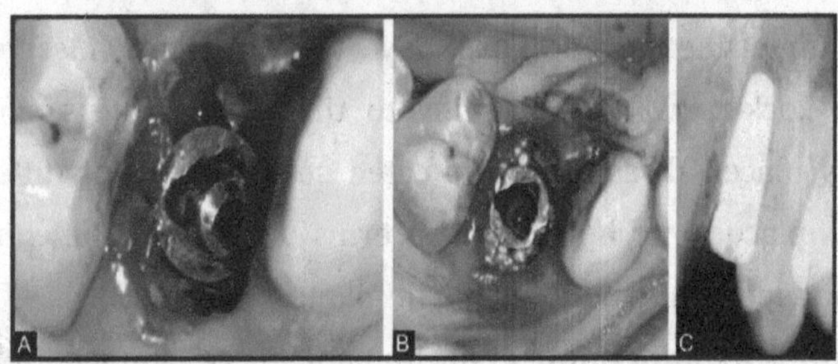

Fig.79 - (A) Immediate implant inserted. (B) Jumping space grafted with an alloplastic, an in situ hardening bone graft substitute (GUIDOR easy-graft CRYSTAL, Sunstar Suisse SA, Etoy, Switzerland). (C) Post implant insertion IOPA.

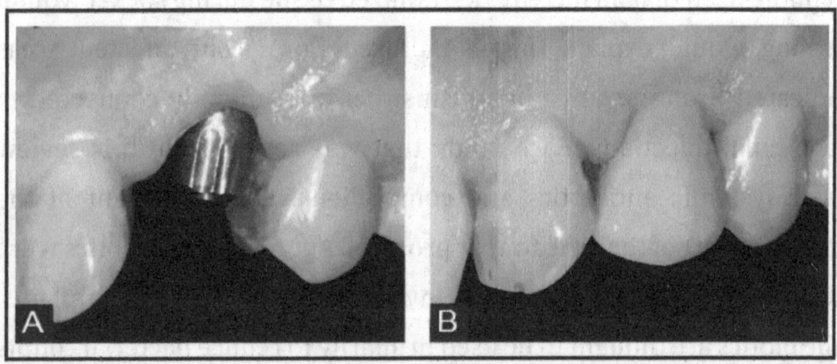

Fig.80 - A) Healed implant with the abutment installed: intraoral view. (B) Final appearance.

In a research, **Kakkar et al.** in **2020,**[168] patients with infected teeth underwent atraumatic extraction of the affected teeth after giving informed consent. The inflammatory, necrotic tissues and pus were thoroughly cleared from sockets by curettage, and extraction sockets were debrided using Er,Cr:YSGG laser (Biolase Technology, Irvine, CA). Immediate implants were placed, and space between socket wall and implant were filled with in situ ,alloplastic hardening bone graft substitute. (GUIDOR easy-graft CRYSTAL, Sunstar Suisse SA, Etoy, Switzerland). **[Fig. 78-80]**

CONCLUSION

The implant success rates achieved by immediate implant placement are comparable to those of conventional protocol, making it a dependable technique. It enables the patient to be much more comfortable, a decrease in the length of time needed for healing, and the preservation of the gingival architecture, which maximizes the visual results. To boost the likelihood of successful clinical parameters ,outcomes, and case selection would be considered.[109]

1. After immediate implant restoration, mean observation period of 19.9 months, there was statistically significant and high incidence recession of buccal marginal mucosa (0.9 0.78mm). Just 14.3% of sites with no recession, whereas 40.5% had at least 1 mm.
2. Sites with implants lingual to this line (1.8 ~ 0.83 vs. 0.6 ~ 0.55mm; P¼0.000) showed 3 times less recession than those in implant buccal to line between cervical margins of neighbouring tooth.
3. In both thick & thin biotype sites, recession was noted, in thin biotype, however, typically had a larger magnitude.
4. The mesial and distal papillae's heights changed very little (mean 0.5mm).

As natural consequence of extraction, additional bone resorption could be avoided with immediate implant implantation. By implanting right away, the ridge collapse process is stopped, protecting the available bone for implant implantation. This method produces more aesthetically pleasing results by preserving both soft tissue and bone. An improved appearance can be achieved with immediate implants by preserving the natural gingival architecture. Because there is no longer a need for a separate healing period following extraction of tooth and implant placement, immediate implant placement shortens duration of overall treatment. For the patient, this may be more practical and comfortable.

Success rates with immediate implant implantation are on par with traditional implant protocols. Implants can be a dependable and predictable treatment for tooth loss if the right cases are chosen, treatment plans are made, and clinical knowledge is applied. Compared to more involved procedures, immediate implant placement is thought to be minimally invasive surgical technique which can result in a quicker recovery and fewer post-operative complications.[169]

REFERENCES

1. Sikri A, Sikri J, Vritti P, Yamika T. Immediate Implant Placement: A Comprehensive Review. Glob J Res Dent Sci. 2023;3:12–24.
2. Becker W, Goldstein M. Immediate implant placement: treatment planning and surgical steps for successful outcome. Periodontol 2000. 2008;47:79–89.
3. Nuzzolese E. Immediate loading of two single tooth implants in the maxilla: preliminary results after one year. J Contemp Dent Pract. 2005;6:148–57.
4. Koh RU, Rudek I, Wang H-L. Immediate implant placement: positives and negatives. Implant Dent. 2010;19:98–108.
5. The glossary of prosthodontic terms: Ninth edition. J Prosthet Dent. 2017;117(5S):e1–105.
6. Gelb DA. Immediate implant surgery: three-year retrospective evaluation of 50 consecutive cases. Int J Oral Maxillofac Implants. 1993;8:388–99.
7. Ring ME. Dentistry: An illustrated history. 1985; Mosby: London, England.
8. Asbell MB. Dentistry: A Historical Perspective: Being a Historical Account of the History of Dentistry from Ancient Times. 1988; Dorrance & Co., Bryn Mawr, Pa.
9. Greenfield EJ. Implantation of artificial crown and bridge abutments. Int J Oral Implantol. 1991;7:63–8.
10. Burch RH. Pinkney Adams - a dentist before his time. Ark Dent. 1997;68:14–5.
11. Linkow LI. Intraosseous implants utilized as fixed bridge

abutments. J Oral Implant Transplant Surg. 1964;10:17–23.

12. Abraham CM. A brief historical perspective on dental implants, their surface coatings and treatments. Open Dent J. 2014; 8:50–5.
13. Brånemark PI, Zarb G, Albrektsson T. Tissue-integrated prostheses: Osseointegration in clinical dentistry. 1985; Quintessence Pub Co Inc.: Chicago.
14. Laney WR. In recognition of an implant pioneer: Professor Dr. André Schroeder. Int J Oral Maxillofac Implants. 1993;8:135–6.
15. Pal T. Fundamentals and history of implant dentistry. J Int Clin Dent Res Organ. 2015;7:6.
16. Alani A, Kelleher M, Bishop K. Peri-implantitis. Part 1: Scope of the problem. Br Dent J. 2014;217:281–7.
17. Bhat S, Kumar A. Biomaterials and bioengineering tomorrow's healthcare. Biomatter. 2013;3:e24717.
18. Kinaia BM, Shah M, Neely AL, Goodis HE. Crestal bone level changes around immediately placed implants: a systematic review and meta-analyses with at least 12 months' follow-up after functional loading. J Periodontol. 2014;85:1537–48.
19. Peeran SW, Ramalingam K. Essentials of Periodontics and Oral Implantology. 1st ed. 2021; Saranraj JPS: Mylapore.
20. Chen ST, Wilson TG Jr, Hämmerle CHF. Immediate or early placement of implants following tooth extraction: review of biologic basis, clinical procedures, and outcomes. Int J Oral Maxillofac Implants. 2004;19 Suppl:12–25.
21. Newman MG, Klokkevold PR, Elangovan S, Kapila Y. Newman and Carranza's clinical periodontology and implantology. 14th

ed. 2023; Saunders: Philadelphia, PA.

22. Esposito M, Grusovin MG, Coulthard P, Worthington HV. Different loading strategies of dental implants: a Cochrane systematic review of randomized controlled clinical trials. Eur J Oral Implantol. 2008 Winter;1:259–76.
23. Funato A, Salama MA, Ishikawa T, Garber DA, Salama H. Timing, positioning, and sequential staging in esthetic implant therapy: a four-dimensional perspective. Int J Periodontics Restorative Dent. 2007;27:313–23.
24. Linkow LI, Chercheve R. Theories and Techniques of Oral Implantalogy. Vol 1. 1970; Mosby: St. Louis.
25. Brånemark P-I, Zarb GA, Albrektsson T. Tissue-integrated prostheses : osseointegration in clinical dentistry. 1985; Quintessence Pub Co Inc: Chicago, IL. p 350.
26. Misch CE. Bone character: second vital implant criterion. Dent Today. 1988; 7:39.
27. Misch CE. Density of bone: effect on treatment planning, surgical approach, and healing. In: Contemporary Implant Dentistry. Misch CE, editor. 1993; Mosby: St. Louis. p 469–85.
28. Misch CE, Kircos LT. Diagnostic imaging and techniques. In: Contemporary Implant Dentistry. 2nd ed. Misch CE, editor. 1999. Mosby: St. Louis; p. 73–87.
29. Albrektsson T, Albrektsson B. Osseointegration of bone implants. A review of an alternative mode of fixation. Acta Orthop Scand. 1987; 58:567–77.
30. Dimitriou R, Babis GC. Biomaterial osseointegration enhancement with biophysical stimulation. J Musculoskelet Neuronal Interact. 2007; 7:253–65.

31. Shetty P, Yadav P, Tahir M, Saini V. Implant design and stress distribution. Int J Oral Implantol Clin Res. 2016; 7:34–9.
32. McGlumphy EA, Peterson LJ, Larsen PE, Jeffcoat MK. Prospective study of 429 hydroxyapatite-coated cylindric omniloc implants placed in 121 patients. Int J Oral Maxillofac Implants. 2003; 18:82–92.
33. Rasmusson L, Kahnberg KE, Tan A. Effects of implant design and surface on bone regeneration and implant stability: an experimental study in the dog mandible. Clin Implant Dent Relat Res. 2001; 3:2–8.
34. Misch CE, Strong JT, Bidez MW. Scientific rationale for dental implant design. In: Dental Implant Prosthetics. Misch CE, editor. 2015; Mosby: St. Louis, MO. p. 340–71.
35. Shreeharsha TV, Sharan S, Brunda K, Pradeep C k., Badola I, Nadira JS. Implant surface modification: A review. Int J Appl Dent Sci. 2020; 6:334–8.
36. Jemat A, Ghazali MJ, Razali M, Otsuka Y. Surface modifications and their effects on titanium dental implants. Biomed Res Int. 2015; 2015:1–11.
37. Ting M, Jefferies SR, Xia W, Engqvist H, Suzuki JB. Classification and effects of implant surface modification on the bone: Human cell-based in vitro studies. J Oral Implantol. 2017; 43:58–83.
38. Cervino G, Fiorillo L, Iannello G, Santonocito D, Risitano G, Cicciù M. Sandblasted and acid etched titanium dental implant surfaces systematic review and confocal microscopy evaluation. Materials (Basel). 2019; 12:1763.
39. Jeong K-I, Kim Y-K, Moon S-W, Kim S-G, Lim S-C, Yun P-Y.

Histologic analysis of resorbable blasting media surface implants retrieved from humans: a report of two cases. J Korean Assoc Oral Maxillofac Surg. 2016; 42:38–42.

40. Alhomsi M. Implications of Titanium Surface Modifications on Dental Implants. EC Dent Sci. 2018; 2064–72.
41. Kumar PS, Ks SK, Grandhi VV, Gupta V. The effects of titanium implant surface topography on osseointegration: Literature review. JMIR Biomed Eng. 2019; 4:13237.
42. Giner L, Mercadé M, Torrent S, Punset M, Pérez RA, Delgado LM, et al. Double acid etching treatment of dental implants for enhanced biological properties. J Appl Biomater Funct Mater. 2018; 16:83–9.
43. Lee J-T, Cho S-A. Biomechanical evaluation of laser-etched Ti implant surfaces vs. chemically modified SLA Ti implant surfaces: Removal torque and resonance frequency analysis in rabbit tibias. J Mech Behav Biomed Mater. 2016; 61:299–307.
44. Kohles SS, Clark MB, Brown CA, Kenealy JN. Direct assessment of profilometric roughness variability from typical implant surface types. Int J Oral Maxillofac Implants. 2004; 19:510–6.
45. Chowdhary R, Mishra S, Kumar M. Anodized dental implant surface. Indian J Dent Res. 2017; 28:76–99.
46. Gotfredsen K, Berglundh T, Lindhe J. Anchorage of titanium implants with different surface characteristics: an experimental study in rabbits. Clin Implant Dent Relat Res. 2000; 2:120–8.
47. Yang Y, Kim K-H, Ong JL. A review on calcium phosphate coatings produced using a sputtering process--an alternative to plasma spraying. Biomaterials. 2005; 26:327–37.

48. Jansen JA, Wolke JG, Swann S, Van der Waerden JP, de Groot K. Application of magnetron sputtering for producing ceramic coatings on implant materials: Magnetron sputtering. Clin Oral Implants Res. 1993; 4:28–34.
49. Bao Q, Chen C, Wang D, Ji Q, Lei T. Pulsed laser deposition and its current research status in preparing hydroxyapatite thin films. Appl Surf Sci. 2005; 252:1538–44.
50. Fernández-Pradas JM, Sardin G, Clèries L, Serra P, Ferrater C, Morenza JL. Deposition of hydroxyapatite thin films by excimer laser ablation. Thin Solid Films. 1998; 317:393–6.
51. Li T, Lee J, Kobayashi T, Aoki H. Hydroxyapatite coating by dipping method, and bone bonding strength. J Mater Sci Mater Med. 1996; 7:355–7.
52. Chai CS, Gross KA, Ben-Nissan B. Critical ageing of hydroxyapatite sol-gel solutions. Biomaterials. 1998; 19:2291–6.
53. Wei M, Ruys AJ, Swain MV, Kim SH, Milthorpe BK, Sorrell CC. Interfacial bond strength of electrophoretically deposited hydroxyapatite coatings on metals. J Mater Sci Mater Med. 1999; 10:401–9.
54. Herø H, Wie H, Jørgensen RB, Ruyter IE. Hydroxyapatite coatings on Ti produced by hot isostatic pressing. J Biomed Mater Res. 1994; 28:343–8.
55. Ohtsuka Y, Matsuura M, Chida N, Yoshinari M, Sumii T, Dérand T. Formation of hydroxyapatite coating on pure titanium substrates by ion beam dynamic mixing. Surf Coat Technol. 1994; 65:224–30.
56. Smeets R, Stadlinger B, Schwarz F, Beck-Broichsitter B, Jung O,

Precht C, et al. Impact of dental implant surface modifications on osseointegration. Biomed Res Int. 2016;1–16

57. Garg H, Bedi G, Garg A. Implant Surface Modifications: A Review. J Clin of Diagn Res. 2012; 6:319–24
58. Webster TJ, Ejiofor JU. Increased osteoblast adhesion on nanophase metals: Ti, Ti6Al4V, and CoCrMo. Biomater. 2004; 25:4731–9.
59. Schliephake H, Scharnweber D, Dard M, Sewing A, Aref A, Roessler S. Functionalization of dental implant surfaces using adhesion molecules. J Biomed Mater Res B Appl Biomater. 2005; 73:88–96.
60. Stigter M, Bezemer J, de Groot K, Layrolle P. Incorporation of different antibiotics into carbonated hydroxyapatite coatings on titanium implants, release and antibiotic efficacy. J Control Release. 2004; 99:127–37.
61. Huang Y-C, Simmons C, Kaigler D, Rice KG, Mooney DJ. Bone regeneration in a rat cranial defect with delivery of PEI-condensed plasmid DNA encoding for bone morphogenetic protein-4 (BMP-4). Gene Ther. 2005; 12:418–26.
62. Beuvelot J, Portet D, Lecollinet G, Moreau M-F, Baslé MF, Chappard D, et al. In vitro kinetic study of growth and mineralization of osteoblast-like cells (Saos-2) on titanium surface coated with a RGD functionalized bisphosphonate. J Biomed Mater Res B Appl Biomater. 2009; 90:873–81.
63. Yeo I-SL. Modifications of dental implant surfaces at the micro- and nano-level for enhanced osseointegration. Materials (Basel). 2019; 13:89.
64. Ma T, Ge X, Zhang Y, Lin Y. Effect of titanium surface

modifications of dental implants on rapid osseointegration. In: Interface Oral Health Science 2016. 2017; Springer: Singapore. p. 247–56.

65. Kalyoncuoglu UT, Yilmaz B, Gungor S. Evaluation of the chitosan-coating effectiveness on a dental titanium alloy in terms of microbial and fibroblastic attachment and the effect of aging. Mater Technol. 2015; 49:925–31.
66. Kaluđerović MR, Schreckenbach JP, Graf H-L. First titanium dental implants with white surfaces: preparation and in vitro tests. Dent Mater. 2014; 30:759–68.
67. Misch CE. Bone character: second vital implant criterion. Dent Today. 1988;7:39–40.
68. Misch CE. Density of bone: effect on treatment plans, surgical approach, healing, and progressive bone loading. Int J Oral Implantol. 1990; 6:23–31.
69. Adell R, Lekholm U, Rockler B, Brånemark P-I. A 15-year study of osseointegrated implants in the treatment of the edentulous jaw. Int J Oral Surg. 1981; 10:387–416.
70. Schnitman PA, Rubenstein JE, Whörle PS, DaSilva JD, Koch GG. Implants for partial edentulism. J Dent Educ. 1988; 52:725–36.
71. Engquist B, Bergendal T, Kallus T, Linden U. A retrospective multicenter evaluation of osseointegrated implants supporting overdentures. Int J Oral Maxillofac Implants. 1988; 3:129–34.
72. Friberg B, Jemt T, Lekholm U. Early failures in 4,641 consecutively placed Brånemark dental implants: a study from stage 1 surgery to the connection of completed prostheses. Int J Oral Maxillofac Implants. 1991; 6:142–6.

73. Jaffin RA, Berman CL. The excessive loss of Branemark fixtures in type IV bone: a 5-year analysis. J Periodontol. 1991; 62:2–4.
74. Johns RB, Jemt T, Heath MR, Hutton JE, McKenna S, McNamara DC, et al. A multicenter study of overdentures supported by Brånemark implants. Int J Oral Maxillofac Implants. 1992; 7:513–22.
75. Smedberg JI, Lothigius E, Bodin I, Frykholm A, Nilner K. A clinical and radiological two-year follow-up study of maxillary overdentures on osseointegrated implants: Maxillary overdentures on osseointegrated implants. Clin Oral Implants Res. 1993; 4:39–46.
76. Snauwaert K, Duyck J, van Steenberghe D, Quirynen M, Naert I. Time dependent failure rate and marginal bone loss of implant supported prostheses: a 15-year follow-up study. Clin Oral Investig. 2000; 4:13–20.
77. Samra RK, Showkat R. Impact of drilling speed in implantology: A review. J Pierre Fauchard Acad. 2021; 35:78–86.
78. Matthews LS, Hirsch C. Temperatures measured in human cortical bone when drilling. J Bone Joint Surg Am. 1972; 54:297–308.
79. Rhinelander FW, Nelson CL, Stewart RD, Stewart CL. Experimental reaming of the proximal femur and acrylic cement implantation: vascular and histologic effects. Clin Orthop Relat Res. 1979; 141:74–89.
80. Thompson HC. Effect of drilling into bone. J Oral Surg (Chic). 1958; 16:22–30.
81. Mishra SK, Chowdhary R. Heat generated by dental implant

drills during osteotomy-a review: heat generated by dental implant drills: Heat generated by dental implant drills. J Indian Prosthodont Soc. 2014; 14:131–43.

82. Oh J-H, Fang Y, Jeong S-M, Choi B-H. The effect of low-speed drilling without irrigation on heat generation: an experimental study. J Korean Assoc Oral Maxillofac Surg. 2016; 142:9–12.
83. Delgado-Ruiz RA, Velasco Ortega E, Romanos GE, Gerhke S, Newen I, Calvo-Guirado JL. Slow drilling speeds for single-drill implant bed preparation. Experimental in vitro study. Clin Oral Investig. 2018; 22:349–59.
84. Watanabe F, Tawada Y, Komatsu S, Hata Y. Heat distribution in bone during preparation of implant sites: heat analysis by real-time thermography. Int J Oral Maxillofac Implants. 1992; 7:212–9.
85. Yacker MJ, Klein M. The effect of irrigation on osteotomy depth and bur diameter. Int J Oral Maxillofac Implants. 1996; 11:634–8.
86. Anitua E. Biological drilling: Implant site preparation in a conservative manner and obtaining autogenous bone grafts. Balkan J Dent Med. 2018; 22:98–101.
87. Hosseinpour S, Tabrizi R, Nazhvanai A, Farahmand M, Pourali S. Do increased drilling speed and depth affect bone viability at implant site? Dent Res J (Isfahan). 2017; 14:331–5.
88. Seo D-U, Kim S-G, Oh J-S, Lim S-C. Comparative study on early osseointegration of implants according to various drilling speeds in the mandible of dogs. Implant Dent. 2017; 26:841–7.

89. Romanos GE, Bastardi DJ, Moore R, Kakar A, Herin Y, Delgado-Ruiz RA. In vitro effect of drilling speed on the primary stability of narrow diameter implants with varying thread designs placed in different qualities of simulated bone. Materials (Basel). 2019; 12:1350.
90. Ozcan M, Salimov F, Temmerman A, Turer OU, Alkaya B, Haytac MC. The evaluation of different osteotomy drilling speed protocols on cortical bone temperature, implant stability and bone healing: An experimental study in an animal model. J Oral Implantol. 2022; 48:3–8.
91. Jeong C-H, Kim D-Y, Shin S-Y, Hong J, Kye S-B, Yang S-M. The effect of implant drilling speed on the composition of particle collected during site preparation. J Korean Acad Periodontol. 2009; 39:253.
92. Tabassum A, Wismeijer D, Hogervorst J, Tahmaseb A. Comparison of proliferation and differentiation of human osteoblast-like cells harvested during implant osteotomy preparation using two different drilling protocols. Int J Oral Maxillofac Implants. 2020; 35:141–9.
93. Kaur G, Tabassum R, Mistry G, Shetty O. Immediate Implant Placement: A Review. J Dent Med Sci. 2017;165:90–5.
94. Beagle JR. Surgical essentials of immediate implant dentistry. 2013. Wiley-Blackwell; Chichester, UK.
95. De Oliveira RR, Macedo GO, Muglia VA, Souza S, Novaes AB, Taba M. Replacement of hopeless retained primary teeth by immediate dental implants: a case report. Int J Oral Maxillofac Implants. 2009; 24:151–4.
96. Becker W, Becker BE, Hujoel P. Retrospective case series

analysis of the factors determining immediate implant placement. Compend Contin Educ Dent. 2000; 21:810–1.

97. Hämmerle C, Araújo MG, Simion M. Evidence-based knowledge on the biology and treatment of extraction sockets. Clin Oral Implants Res. 2011; 23:80–2.
98. Dawson A, Chen S. The SAC Classification in Implant Dentistry. 2009. Quintessence Pub Co Inc: New Malden, England.
99. Hämmerle C, Stone P, Jung RE, Kapos T, Brodala N. Consensus statements and recommended clinical procedures regarding computer-assisted implant dentistry. Int J Oral Maxillofac Implants. 2009; 24:126–31.
100. Mayfield L, Nobréus N, Attström R, Linde A. Guided bone regeneration in dental implant treatment using a bioabsorbable membrane. Clin Oral Implants Res. 1997; 8:10–7.
101. Buser D, von Arx T, ten Bruggenkate C, Weingart D. Basic surgical principles with ITI implants. Clin Oral Implants Res. 2000; 11:59–68.
102. Fugazzotto PA, De Paoli S. Sinus floor augmentation on at the time of maxillary molar extraction: Success and failure rates of 137 implants in function for up to 3 years. J Periodontol. 2002; 73:39–44.
103. Buser D, Chen ST, Weber HP, Belser UC. Early implant placement following single-tooth extraction in the esthetic zone: biologic rationale and surgical procedures. Int J Periodontics Restorative Dent. 2008; 28:441–51.
104. Belser UC, Buser D, Hämmerle C, Jung R, Martin WC, Morton D, et al. Implant Therapy in the Esthetic Zone: Single-Tooth

Replacements. In: ITI Treatment Guide Volume 1. Buser D, Belser U, Wismeijer D, editors. 2019. Quintessence Pub Co Inc: New Malden, England.

105. Kois JC. Predictable single-tooth peri-implant esthetics: five diagnostic keys. Compend Contin Educ Dent. 2004; 25:895–6, 898, 900 passim; quiz 906–7.
106. Rupprecht RD, Horning GM, Nicoll BK, Cohen ME. Prevalence of dehiscences and fenestrations in modern American skulls. J Periodontol. 2001; 72:722–9.
107. Buser D, Wittneben J, Bornstein MM, Grütter L, Chappuis V, Belser UC. Stability of contour augmentation and esthetic outcomes of implant-supported single crowns in the esthetic zone: 3-year results of a prospective study with early implant placement postextraction. J Periodontol. 2011; 82:342–9.
108. Morton D, Chen ST, Martin WC, Levine RA, Buser D. Consensus statements and recommended clinical procedures regarding optimizing esthetic outcomes in implant dentistry. Int J Oral Maxillofac Implants. 2014;29 Suppl:216–20.
109. Amine M, El Kholti W, Laalou Y, Bennani A, Kissa J. Immediate Implant Placement: A Review. J Dent Forecast. 2018; 1: 1013.
110. Meijer HJA, Raghoebar GM. Immediate implant placement in molar extraction sites: a 1-year prospective case series pilot study. Int J Implant Dent. 2020; 6.
111. Slagter KW, Raghoebar GM, Hentenaar DFM, Vissink A, Meijer HJA. Immediate placement of single implants with or without immediate provisionalization in the maxillary aesthetic region: A 5-year comparative study. J Clin Periodontol. 2021; 48:272–83.

112. Garcia-Sanchez R, Mardas N, Buti J, Ortiz Ruiz AJ, Pardo Zamora G. Immediate implant placement in fresh alveolar sockets with a minimal split-thickness envelope flap: A randomised controlled clinical trial. Clin Oral Implants Res. 2021; 32:1115–26.
113. Crippa R, Aiuto R, Dioguardi M, Nieri M, Peñarrocha-Diago M, Peñarrocha-Diago M, et al. Immediate dental implant placement in post-extraction-infected sites decontaminated with Er,Cr:YSGG laser: a retrospective cohort study. Odontology. 2023; 111:255–62.
114. Hirani M, Moshtofar Z, Devine M, Paolinelis G, Djemal S. Survival of immediate implants replacing traumatised teeth in the anterior maxilla. Br Dent J. 2023.
115. Çolak S, Demïrsoy MS. Retrospective analysis of dental implants immediately placed in extraction sockets with periapical pathology: immediate implant placement in infected areas. BMC Oral Health. 2023; 23.
116. Bambini F, Memè L, Rossi R, Grassi A, Grego S, Mummolo S. New operative protocol for immediate post-extraction implant in lower-first-molar region with Rex-blade implants: A case series with 18 months of follow-up. Appl Sci (Basel). 2023;13:10226.
117. Bahaa A, Bahaa AM, El-Bagoury N, Khaled N, Ibrahim AM. Immediate implants in posterior extraction sites: A case series applying the dual-zone therapeutic concept with a three-year follow-up. Cureus. 2024;16:e54890.
118. Dhami B, Shrestha P, Gupta S, Pandey N. Immediate Implant Placement: Current Concepts. J Nepal Soc Perio Oral

Implantology. 2019; 3:18–24.

119. Chen ST, Darby IB, Reynolds EC. A prospective clinical study of non-submerged immediate implants: clinical outcomes and aesthetic results. Clin Oral Implants Res. 2007; 18:552–62.
120. Guéhennec L, Soueidan L, Layrolle A, Amouriq P. Surface treatments of titanium dental implants for rapid osseointegration. Dent Mater. 2007; 23:844–54.
121. Huwais S, Meyer E. A novel osseous densification approach in implant osteotomy preparation to increase biomechanical primary stability, bone mineral density, and bone-to-implant contact. Int J Oral Maxillofac Implants. 2017;32:27–36.
122. Huwais S, inventor; Huwais IP Holding LLC, assignee. Fluted osteotome and surgical method for use. United States patent. 2020 US 10,568,639.
123. Bleyan S, Huwais S, Neiva R. Osseodensification effective for immediate molar replacement. Compend Contin Educ Dent. 2022; 43:444–52.
124. Trisi P, Berardini M, Falco A, Podaliri Vulpiani M. New osseodensification implant site preparation method to increase bone density in low-density bone: In vivo evaluation in sheep. Implant Dent. 2016;25:24–31.
125. Ibrahim A, Ayad S, ElAshwah A. The effect of osseodensification technique on implant stability (clinical trial). Alex Dent J. 2020;45:1–7.
126. Bergamo ETP, Zahoui A, Barrera RB, Huwais S, Coelho PG, Karateew ED, et al. Osseodensification effect on implants primary and secondary stability: Multicenter controlled clinical trial. Clin Implant Dent Relat Res. 2021;23:317–28.

127. Stacchi C, Troiano G, Montaruli G, Mozzati M, Lamazza L, Antonelli A, et al. Changes in implant stability using different site preparation techniques: Osseodensification drills versus piezoelectric surgery. A multi-center prospective randomized controlled clinical trial. Clin Implant Dent Relat Res. 2023;25:133–40.
128. Costa JA, Mendes JM, Salazar F, Pacheco JJ, Rompante P, Moreira JF, et al. Osseodensification vs. Conventional osteotomy: A case series with cone beam computed tomography. J Clin Med. 2024;13:1568.
129. Bhola M, Neely AL, Kolhatkar S. Immediate implant placement: clinical decisions, advantages, and disadvantages. J Prosthodont. 2008; 17:576–81.
130. Resnik R. Misch's contemporary implant dentistry. 4th ed. 2020; Mosby: St. Louis, MO.
131. Lin G-H, Chan H-L, Bashutski JD, Oh T-J, Wang H-L. The effect of flapless surgery on implant survival and marginal bone level: a systematic review and meta-analysis. J Periodontol. 2014; 85:e91-103.
132. Campelo LD, Camara JRD. Flapless implant surgery: a 10-year clinical retrospective analysis. Int J Oral Maxillofac Implants. 2002; 17:271–6.
133. Rocci A, Martignoni M, Gottlow J. Immediate loading in the maxilla using flapless surgery, implants placed in predetermined positions, and prefabricated provisional restorations: a retrospective 3-year clinical study. Clin Implant Dent Relat Res. 2003; 5:29–36.
134. Stefanini M, Rendón A, Zucchelli A, Sangiorgi M, Zucchelli G.

Avoiding errors and complications related to immediate implant placement in the esthetic area with a mucogingival approach. Periodontol 2000. 2023;92:362–72.

135. Wagenberg BD, Froum SJ. Implant complications related to immediate implant placement into extraction sites. In: Froum SJ, editor. Dental Implant Complications: Etiology, Prevention, and Treatment. Chicester, UK: Wiley-Blackwell; 2015. p. 457–80.
136. Chen ST, Buser D, Sculean A, Belser UC. Complications and treatment errors in implant positioning in the aesthetic zone: Diagnosis and possible solutions. Periodontol 2000. 2023;92:220–34.
137. Buser D, Martin W, Belser UC. Optimizing esthetics for implant restorations in the anterior maxilla: anatomic and surgical considerations. Int J Oral Maxillofac Implants. 2004;19:43–61.
138. Wismeijer D, Chen S, Buser D, editors. ITI treatment guide, volume 10: Implant therapy in the esthetic zone: Current treatment modalities and materials for single-tooth replacements. In Berlin, Germany: Quintessenz Verlags; 2017. p. 357.
139. Zigdon H, Machtei EE. The dimensions of keratinized mucosa around implants affect clinical and immunological parameters. Clin Oral Implants Res. 2008;19:387–92.
140. Schrott AR, Jimenez M, Hwang J-W, Fiorellini J, Weber H-P. Five-year evaluation of the influence of keratinized mucosa on peri-implant soft-tissue health and stability around implants supporting full-arch mandibular fixed prostheses. Clin Oral Implants Res. 2009;20:1170–7.

141. Boynueğri D, Nemli SK, Kasko YA. Significance of keratinized mucosa around dental implants: a prospective comparative study. Clin Oral Implants Res. 2013;24:928–33.
142. Lang NP, Löe H. The relationship between the width of keratinized gingiva and gingival health. J Periodontol. 1972;43:623–7.
143. Kungsadalpipob K, Supanimitkul K, Manopattanasoontorn S, Sophon N, Tangsathian T, Arunyanak SP. The lack of keratinized mucosa is associated with poor peri-implant tissue health: a cross-sectional study. Int J Implant Dent. 2020;6:28.
144. Souza AB, Tormena M, Matarazzo F, Araújo MG. The influence of peri-implant keratinized mucosa on brushing discomfort and peri-implant tissue health. Clin Oral Implants Res. 2016;27:650–5.
145. Grunder U, Gracis S, Capelli M. Influence of the 3-D bone-to-implant relationship on esthetics. Int J Periodontics Restorative Dent. 2005;25:113–9.
146. Chen ST, Buser D. Clinical and esthetic outcomes of implants placed in postextraction sites. Int J Oral Maxillofac Implants. 2009;24:186–217.
147. Crespi R, Capparè P, Gherlone E. A 4-year evaluation of the Peri-implant parameters of immediately loaded implants placed in fresh extraction sockets. J Periodontol. 2010;81:1629–34.
148. Juodzbalys G, Bojarskas S, Kubilius R, Wang H-L. Using the support immersion endoscope for socket assessment. J Periodontol. 2008;79:64–71.

149. Mayfield L. Immediate, delayed and late submerged and transmucosal implants. In: Lang NP, Karring T, Lindhe J, editors. Proceedings of the Third European Workshop on Periodontology Implant Dentistry. Berlin: Quintessenz; 1999. p. 520–34.
150. Kourtis SG, Sotiriadou S, Voliotis S, Challas A. Private practice results of dental implants. Part I: Survival and evaluation of risk factors—part II: Surgical and prosthetic complications. Implant Dent. 2004;13:373–85.
151. Kochar SP, Reche A, Paul P. The etiology and management of dental implant failure: A review. Cureus. 2022;10:e30455.
152. Thoma DS, Gil A, Hämmerle CHF, Jung RE. Management and prevention of soft tissue complications in implant dentistry. Periodontol 2000. 2022; 88:116–29.
153. van Kesteren CJ, Schoolfield J, West J, Oates T. A prospective randomized clinical study of changes in soft tissue position following immediate and delayed implant placement. Int J Oral Maxillofac Implants. 2010; 25:562–70.
154. Lang NP, Pun L, Lau KY, Li KY, Wong MCM. A systematic review on survival and success rates of implants placed immediately into fresh extraction sockets after at least 1 year. Clin Oral Implants Res. 2012; 23:39–66.
155. Bianchi AE, Sanfilippo F. Single-tooth replacement by immediate implant and connective tissue graft: a 1-9-year clinical evaluation. Clin Oral Implants Res. 2004; 15:269–77.
156. Lee C, Tao C, Stoupel J. The Effect of Subepithelial Connective Tissue Graft Placement on Esthetic Outcomes Following Immediate Implant Placement: Systematic Review. J

Periodontol. 2016; 87:156–67.

157. Canullo L, Iurlaro G, Iannello G. Double-blind randomized controlled trial study on post-extraction immediately restored implants using the switching platform concept: soft tissue response. Preliminary report. Clin Oral Implants Res. 2009; 20:414–20.

158. Bruno V, O'Sullivan D, Badino M, Catapano S. Preserving soft tissue after placing implants in fresh extraction sockets in the maxillary esthetic zone and a prosthetic template for interim crown fabrication: a prospective study. J Prosthet Dent. 2014; 111:195–202.

159. Kaur J, Chahal GS, Grover V, Bansal D, Jain A. Immediate implant placement in periodontally infected sites - A systematic review and meta-analysis. J Int Acad Periodontol. 2021; 23:115-137.

160. Casap N, Zeltser C, Wexler A, Tarazi E, Zeltser R. Immediate placement of dental implants into debrided infected dentoalveolar sockets. J Oral Maxillofac Surg. 2007; 65:384–92.

161. Quirynen M, Gijbels F, Jacobs R. An infected jawbone site compromising successful osseointegration. Periodontol 2000. 2003; 33:129–44.

162. Alsaadi G, Quirynen M, Komárek A, van Steenberghe D. Impact of local and systemic factors on the incidence of oral implant failures, up to abutment connection. J Clin Periodontol. 2007; 34:610–7.

163. Pecora G, Andreana S, Covani U, De Leonardis D, Schifferle RE. New directions in surgical endodontics; immediate

implantation into an extraction site. J Endod. 1996; 22:135–9.

164. Anitua E, Piñas L, Alkhraisat MH. Long-term outcomes of immediate implant placement into infected sockets in association with immediate loading: A retrospective cohort study. J Periodontol. 2016; 87:1135–40.
165. Zuffetti F, Capelli M, Galli F, Del Fabbro M, Testori T. Post-extraction implant placement into infected versus non-infected sites: A multicenter retrospective clinical study. Clin Implant Dent Relat Res. 2017; 19:833–40.
166. Novaes AB Jr, Marcaccini AM, Souza SLS, Taba M Jr, Grisi MFM. Immediate placement of implants into periodontally infected sites in dogs: a histomorphometric study of bone-implant contact. Int J Oral Maxillofac Implants. 2003; 18:391–8.
167. Lindeboom JAH, Tjiook Y, Kroon FHM. Immediate placement of implants in periapical infected sites: a prospective randomized study in 50 patients. Oral Surg Oral Med Oral Pathol Oral Radiol Endod. 2006; 101:705–10.
168. Kakar A, Kakar K, Leventis MD, Jain G. Immediate implant placement in infected sockets: A consecutive cohort study. J Lasers Med Sci. 2020; 11:167–73.
169. Evans CDJ, Chen ST. Esthetic outcomes of immediate implant placements. Clin Oral Implants Res. 2008; 19:73-80

www.ingramcontent.com/pod-product-compliance
Lightning Source LLC
LaVergne TN
LVHW031426170726
843492LV00009B/2874

* 9 7 8 8 1 9 7 7 9 2 7 2 4 *